BEYOND GENTLE TEACHING

A Nonaversive Approach to
Helping Those in Need

BEYOND GENTLE TEACHING

A Nonaversive Approach to Helping Those in Need

John J. McGee
and
Frank J. Menolascino
Creighton University Medical Center
Omaha, Nebraska

PLENUM PRESS • NEW YORK AND LONDON

Library of Congress Cataloging in Publication Data

McGee, John J.
 Beyond gentle teaching: a nonaversive approach to helping those in need / John J.
McGee and Frank J. Menolascino.
  p.   cm.
 Includes bibliographical references and index.
 ISBN 0-306-43856-9
 1. Social work with the handicapped. I. Menolascino, Frank J., date. II. Title.
HV1553.M39 1991   91-14502
362.3′8 – dc20   CIP

ISBN 0-306-43856-9

© 1991 Plenum Press, New York
A Division of Plenum Publishing Corporation
233 Spring Street, New York, N.Y. 10013

Printed in the United States of America

PREFACE

This book is for caregivers: those who care for and about children and adults who reside on the very edge of family and community life. It is for those who not only want to help these distanced individuals but for those who also want to change themselves in the process. It is for parents, teachers, direct care workers, counselors, social workers, psychologists, psychiatrists, advocates, and all who strive to bring about just treatment for the marginalized. It is for those who want to consider a psychology based on interdependence and to uncover ways to express and practice companionship instead of control. It is about children and adults who live in marginalized conditions, who are pushed and pulled away from feelings of union and hurt themselves, hurt others, or simply give up. It is for those who live and work among the mentally retarded, the mentally ill, the aged, the homeless, and the poor. To be marginalized is to be easily controlled, isolated, and segregated. And being a caregiver is more than just caring; it is entering into a mutual change process with the person by becoming more of a human being instead of less—the parent embracing the crying child instead of yelling at him, the teacher befriending a lonely child instead of punishing her, the psychiatric nurse sitting with the confused and belligerent patient instead of closing the heavy seclusion room door, the social worker creating circles of friends around the homeless person instead of simply dishing out soup.

This book has emerged out of our experiences with children and adults with severe behavioral difficulties and represents a new way of thinking about our role with persons in need. It presents a new psychology—one based on mutual change, the establishment of feelings of companionship, and an array of strategies and techniques to bring about interactional change.

It breaks away from the current trend in psychology that uses a two-edged system of reward and punishment to change disruptive or destructive behaviors. Many, if not most, of the practices related to mental health, mental retardation, social services, and parenting are based on behaviorism. For those who cling to the edge of family and community life, this means earning reward or receiving punishment. This approach might work for some. It might make the aggressive meek, the loud quiet, the disruptive complacent, and the disobedient compliant. However, we are not interested in changing only the other person. We have tried to develop a process that helps to change both ourselves and others—a psychology of interdependence. In many respects, behaviorism and behavior modification have had their day. Institutions, jails, and shelters are filled with thousands of those who have been modified; yet their faces tell another story—one of meaninglessness, aloneness, and lack of choice. This book is intended to share with caregivers an option—one that helps bring meaning, feelings of companionship, and a fuller life to ourselves and those whom we serve.

In this book, we present a psychology of interdependence that asks us to change together along with those whom we are serving. It places unconditional valuing at the center of the caregiving and therapeutic process. It does not wait for those who are marginalized to earn reward, but offers valuing without question and with the hope of transformation. It puts aside compliance as a central purpose and replaces it with the establishment of feelings of companionship.

This book examines our values and invites us to move toward a culture of life instead of violence. We examine a number of supportive ways to bring this about. We have tried to make this book as practical as possible, but also to share with caregivers a framework for reflection and questioning. It is not a quick solution to complex personal, interpersonal, and societal problems; it is the beginning of a journey toward interdependence.

John J. McGee
Frank J. Menolascino

Omaha, Nebraska

CONTENTS

ix

Chapter 1
INTERDEPENDENCE
The Fulfillment of Being with Others

Introduction

Interdependence is a way of looking at ourselves and those who cling to the slippery edges of family and community life. It views us and others as equals, as a people who long for companionship, as a people in pain, and as a people who struggle for human rights and hunger for unity. It is a life-long project that brings about healing in us and those whom we serve and calls on us to confirm and express our solidarity with others. Interdependence involves purposes different from those that are typically thought of. Instead of focusing on getting rid of aggression or self-injury and worrying about compliance or obedience, interdependence calls on us to teach new ways of interacting. Instead of seeing ourselves as those who control, we struggle to create community. Interdependence leads us to bring about feelings of union, emotional well-being, and the instillation of hope at the center of our lives and of those whom we serve.

Yet, in reality we find that this is not always the case. Caregiving becomes overpowering, the strong are bent on controlling the weak, obedience takes the place of companionship. Independence holds more sway than interdependence.

Kathleen has been homeless, but is now in a state institution. Her schizophrenia has left her confused, aggressive, and obstinate. Her homelessness has left her hopeless. She stands at the far end of the asylum's corridor. A caregiver approaches, it is time to do an

1

activity. She could care less. The caregiver tells her to come. She yells and slaps him. She feels nothing but fear. To her, his words conjure up force, and his hands are like weapons. And he stands there, angry as the slap stings his face and her loud screams echo down the hallway. He grabs her. She rips off her blouse and then her pants. Her trembling hands gouge at her rectum. She feels no choice but to hurt herself and attack her aggressor. Soon the ward's loudspeaker is summoning, "All staff!" Two strong aides arrive; they hold Kathleen's arms and bring her to the floor where she is to remain for two minutes or until she calms down. Yet she fights more. Their hands tighten their grip. Finally she quiets, she has been subdued. One of the caregivers says, "Good girl! Now you go to the recreation area." She stands up with her head bowed and accompanies them. Compliance has been victorious.

These caregivers opted for control, and they had enough strength to bring it about. However, we need to ask ourselves, "What kind of feelings do these caregivers represent?" and "What must Kathleen see in them?"

We have two options: to control Kathleen through force by using restraint and punishment, or to establish a feeling of union by unconditionally valuing her while weathering the storms of change. A spirit of interdependence leads us to view Kathleen in the light of an evolving feeling of companionship and to commit ourselves to actions that help to free us as well as her. We would not look at her as a client who needs to learn to comply or needs to learn a lesson in obedience, but as a woman who, like everybody else, is in the process of learning to live with others and find fulfillment in them. We need to acknowledge her seeming desire to remain apart, but also affirm and enable a sense of coming together. Rather than get into an emotional or physical tug-of-war, her caregiver needs to decide to teach her to feel safe and secure, enable her to feel that it is good to be engaged and participate with others, and teach her that unconditional valuing is at the center of the human condition. At the worst moments, she needs to receive the most valuing and enter into a process of learning to live in friendship, a relationship that finds its origins in the unconditional recognition of her worth and wholeness as well as our own. Where does this leave us with Kathleen? Is it possible to enter into her fearful and disconnected world with warmth and valuing instead of coldness and contingencies? Is an emerging feeling of companionship possible?

Another caregiver has decided to establish a different relationship with Kathleen—one based on feelings of their interdependence and expressed through unconditional valuing. Later in the day, he sees Kathleen in the day room. She has been placed in a restraint chair with her arms and legs strapped down. He walks up to her and touches her hand. His face expresses kindness. His hands signal warmth. His words speak of friendship. Of course, Kathleen has no reason to trust him. She spits in his face, but he pays this no heed; instead he loosens the straps and continues talking to her. She screams, "Want restraints!" but he drops them to the floor. He realizes that his kind and soothing words will initially fall on deaf ears and will not penetrate her hardened heart, but he also recognizes that he needs to endure her onslaughts and represent safety and security. He says, "Kathleen, I know that you are afraid. But together we can go to the activity room. I will stay with you."

The other caregivers gawk at him and say, "You're going to have to take her by the arms! She's dangerous." He ignores their mockery and touches her hand. She recoils, but he perseveres, "You know what friends do? Shake hands! Don't worry though, I will not force you to do anything. I will just stay with you." She lets him touch her hands for a second and looks up at him. She then jumps up and runs to a corner. He accompanies her and continues to dialogue with her. She flails her arms at him, but he continues to reach out and speak kindly to her. The minutes wear on. She makes more attempts at slapping, screaming, and running away.

At one point, she sits in a corner and rocks. He sits on the floor next to her and reaches out his hand. She does nothing. He tries to express nurturing and warmth, but she seems unresponsive. Yet he realizes that the longer she tarries with him the safer she is feeling. He reaches more closely and she lets him touch her hand. However, in the next instant, her hand reaches inside her pants.

She screams and closes her eyes. The caregiver thinks, "Will she ever move toward me?" He checks his cynicism and seeks deeply for his values. He reaches his hand out again. Kathleen looks at it and then at him. She removes her hand from her crotch and lets him pat her on the back. The caregiver knows that this simple act of reaching out is the mere beginning of an inching toward a new relationship. He realizes that if their mutuality is to evolve, he will need to persevere with her, and she will gradually move toward him in an ebb and flow.

A PSYCHOLOGY OF INTERDEPENDENCE

A psychology of human interdependence concerns itself with the whole being—mind, body, emotions, and spirit—not just observable behavior, but also the inner nature of the human condition. It focuses on the marginalized person as well as the caregiver. It is a process that breaks us from the chains of control through a coming together with those who are marginalized. It brings us and others into a process of solidarity. But it needs to start with *us*. We are the ones who have to initiate it. It calls for transformation in our inner lives, the way we see ourselves and others, and the recognition that unfolding interdependence is a vital and central dimension of our life condition. It has to do with our initial recognition of our values and practices and the need for us to change before we consider other' behaviors. It is based on the belief that all of us long to be companions in this life and that this feeling for being with others and a sense of belonging resides in all of us.

Yet, why is it that some individuals hit, kick, scream, spit, and hurt themselves? Why is it that others withdraw into isolation or seek meaning in the loneliness of the streets. Why is it that some fall into the depths of despair or mental disorganization? Could it be that this longing does not exist? Regardless of the type of aggression, self-injury, or withdrawal, we assume that a hunger for being with others rests in the human spirit, longs to be fulfilled, and, in many instances, needs to be discovered. We struggle to discover and fulfill this need in ourselves and others. We are often

Interdependence is

- The recognition of our own and others' wholeness—mind, body, emotions, and spirit
- The affirmation of the worth of all people, the marginalized and the opulent
- The assumption that all long for feelings of relatedness and being at home with others
- The need to accept, understand, and empathize with the human condition of marginalized others
- The critical questioning and rejection of values and practices that seek to control and dominate
- The recognition of caregiving as a means of promoting personal and social change—transforming ourselves and others
- The centering of all interactions on unconditional valuing
- The commitment to struggle for a culture of life and social justice
- A political act based on solidarity with others

pushed by the fear of giving ourselves to others and, at the same time, pulled by the hope that such feelings give rise to. Our fear can lead us to lord over others in order to gain a false sense of power. But the more we question our values, the more our hope can lead us to feelings of companionship. This pushing and pulling leaves us in a quandary: to reach out toward others or to preside over them. The desire to affirm the other is often buried in us by years of training that have taught us that independence is the central goal of life and that, for those who are on the fringes of community, compliance is the pathway to success. Yet self-reliance and blind obedience are lonely conditions that lock us and others out of the embrace of human warmth and affection. Those who are committed to caregiving often do not recognize this struggle within themselves, let alone in the marginalized people whom they serve. So the first place to start in a psychology of interdependence is with ourselves, our values, and how we translate these into reality.

A psychology of interdependence calls for a different perspective than what is typically seen in caregiving. Humanistic psychology speaks of the glory of individualism and the striving for personal peak experiences. Interdependence, even though it facilitates and honors self-development, goes beyond the walls of the person and calls for the pursuit of social justice. It asks us to see and help heal personal realities and also the unjust social conditions that often surround human anguish: the abandonment of institutions, the loneliness of psychiatric ghettoes, the tragedy of homelessness. Behaviorism looks at humans as machine-like entities, responding to the power of reward for deeds well done and punishment for their absence. Interdependence recognizes a basic need for relatedness and assumes that this longing transcends the self and is more important then rote obedience. It puts aside the drive for individualism and the attitude that everyone should lift themselves up by his or her own bootstraps. It recognizes and clarifies the vulnerabilities within the human condition, and especially embraces those who live marginalized lives due to disabilities, mental illness, poverty, and racism.

Origins of a Psychology of Interdependence

This psychology's origins evolved from our work among marginalized people in the Americas. The slum dwellers of northeastern Brazil taught us much, for in the Third World interdependence is a necessary way of life, where absolute poverty drives people to help or seek help from one another and where the people recognize that a culture of life and a culture of death are posed in an omnipresent battle. This struggle necessarily rejects domination and seeks freedom, not just for self, but for all. In working among the children of prostitutes and thousands of other street children in a city called Juazeiro, it became clear that education and psychology need to reach out to those in pain, and that this act not only helps to liberate the other person, but frees those who are working with others. Some of these children were handicapped. Some had no parents. All lived on the street, under bridges, in gutters, and in cardboard shanties. Yet even these little ones strived to help one another, sharing bread crumbs, filthy water, and tattered blankets. These children fought to survive and found solace in themselves. They knew that their existence depended on their friends.

It was paradoxical to enter the institutions of North America and find another Third World in the midst of bounty—institutions where the mentally retarded, the aged, and the mentally ill were subjected to control and compliance as if these were the be-all and end-all of the human condition. Then and now, it is virtually impossible to enter an institution for those who are old, infirm, mentally ill, or mentally retarded and not smell the wretched odors, not see the empty eyes, and not be touched by the cringing bodies. It is astonishing to walk North America's streets, walled in by riches, and see the countless numbers of homeless people, with their ghostly faces expressing the same hopelessness as those who are institutionalized. It is difficult to pass through special schools where the handicapped, the behaviorally disordered, and the "failures" sit silently awaiting unknown and empty independence. And it is equally difficult to walk through many programs that are in the community, but not of it—with locked doors, rules, isolation, and loneliness.

Through our work among thousands of children and adults in these settings, it became clear that psychology needed to reflect a different spirit and purpose. This was brought home when we began to help establish community programs for the mentally retarded in the early 1970s. We soon learned that being in the community did not necessarily mean being of it. The probability of social integration was increased, but not assured. Roofs over heads and food on the table in a neighborhood did not guarantee feelings of being with others. At the same time, behavior modification had appeared as the technology for caregivers to use in these settings. Soon control was the norm and compliance was the purpose. The lives of those marginalized people became centered on reward and punishment. Verbal reward and reprimands took the place of conversation. Time-out rooms were located next

Gentle teaching is
- The first step in creating feelings of companionship
- A set of strategies that encourages unconditional valuing and human engagement
- An approach that calls for mutual transformation
- An ongoing way of interacting
- A prelude to a psychology of interdependence

to living rooms and physical restraint replaced warm embraces. As the years have gone by, such practices have become more professionalized, systematic, and sophisticated. And the marginalized person has become lost in a maze of individualized plans which are depersonalized, enchanted with control and consequences.

In response to these experiences and realities, we developed gentle teaching. This was initially an approach that gave us and other caregivers an alternative to punishment practices. It soon taught us that change in the other does not come about without change in ourselves. Our values and beliefs are critical elements, and finding ways to express them has transformed gentle teaching from a supportive approach into a psychology of interdependence. Thousands of people like Kathleen and their caregivers have taught us that we can break away from control and consequences, and to do this we need to articulate and practice human interdependence.

Our experiences with gentle teaching have taught us that change needs to start with ourselves. We need to exude warmth, be tolerant, and translate our values into relationships based on companionship. Our interactions need to reflect warm caring and a spirit of oneness in spite of even intense rejection or rebellion. They need to begin to signal feelings of empathy and the understanding that the relationship will evolve into an authentic friendship even though initially it is quite lopsided. Our interactions need to center on valuing the person with unconditional respect during the best moments and the most difficult ones. We have to care about and express our support for the person. Spit could be running down our face or slaps stinging our arms, but we need to unconditionally value the other. We are asked to transmit this feeling through dialogue and sharing our life experiences with the other. Our task is to initiate this process in a spirit of human solidarity. Warmth can be felt in the tone of our voice, the sincerity of our gaze, and the serenity of our movements. Tolerance is conveyed through patience in the face of aggression, respect in the face of rejection, and perseverance in the face of entrenched rebellion. Our values are the impetus within this process, and they need to be constantly questioned and deepened. It is this spirit that we have learned in our gentle teaching experiences—learning to break away from emotional homelessness, rupture the cold grip of loneliness, and center ourselves on unconditional valuing.

The challenge is not to find nonaversive behavioral techniques, but to formulate and put into practice a psychology of interdependence that goes against the grain of modifying the other and asks for mutual change. This presents a major challenge to parents, professionals, and advocates. It requires an awakening of our values and putting them into practice in the most difficult situations.

> Patrick is a 6-year-old boy who has his loving parents and teacher almost pulling out their hair. At home and school, he is a terror, throwing everything in sight onto the floor, tantruming, hitting, scratching, and spitting in their faces when nothing else seems to insult them. He has become the school's "spitter," and everyone knows him by that name. When extremely mad, his last resort is to insult anyone asking him to do anything with a sally of spit. He knows that this is the last straw. The teacher calls the mother almost every morning to pick him up due to his extreme disruptiveness. The mother endures the same behavior at home. The family is at its wit's end and is about to send him to a special live-in school for disturbed children. They have been nurturing, affectionate, and warm toward him, yet he acts as though they are his enemies.

How can these caregivers reach Patrick and help him feel at home? First, they need to look at themselves. More than simply ignoring these behaviors and redirecting him so that they can reward him, his caregivers need to express ongoing warmth and unconditional valuing. They have to find ways to protect him and others without domineering him. They need to enable him to feel that it is good to be with them. At the same time, they have to look at the subtle ways in which they signal fear and demands and dramatically decrease any expressions of coldness and superiority.

His mother and father think about this possibility: increasing their valuing, making sure that it is unconditional, and also seeking to draw it from him. They realize that it will be a long and energy-consuming process, but perhaps worth it. That morning, the mother sits with her son in the kitchen. He is bawling and screaming. The mother has some silverware and a tray on the table and wants to use this to structure the time. Patrick wants nothing to do with sitting there, doing a task, or just being with his mother. She feels horrible about this rejection that is like rubbing salt more deeply into her emotional wound; yet she has decided to teach him that he is safe with her. Her hands and words will not signal violence or force; rather, they will represent valuing and doing things together.

Patrick's parents and teacher went through this questioning process and persevered with him. He slowly began to accept and even seek out being with them, his brothers and sisters, and schoolmates.

In the first days, Patrick's friends and family fight against the urge to control and dominate him. He does everything he can to shove them away physically and emotionally. But as the spit flies from his mouth and lands right on his teacher's face, she continues to give him value and focus on the goodness of being together. As the week progresses, the mother and teacher feel slightly more at ease and start to ask for hugs. And, after an hour of screaming, tossing objects, and spitting, he runs toward his mother, smiles, and embraces her. She feels relieved and senses that they are on the road to a different relationship. Yet, like Kathleen's caregiver, she and the teacher recognize that this will be a difficult process and that they will need to endure more onslaughts.

Change in Patrick means change in his caregiver. Gentle teaching has taught us many of the supportive techniques that can help us avoid punishment and highlight ourselves as rewarding people. A psychology of interdependence helps us put companionship at the heart of the purpose of the caregiving so that we enter into a new relationship with others.

COMPANIONSHIP: THE PURPOSE OF CAREGIVING

The instillation of feelings of companionship calls on us to express warmth to those who are cold, affection to those who are emptied of feeling, tolerance of those why try to harm us, and authenticity to those who are constantly subjected to sterile programs. As caregivers, our first task is to initiate a process in which we and marginalized others learn to accept and express valuing. The initial commitment falls on us; otherwise the other is left unable to reach out. It begins in a one-to-one relationship that at first places us in a most difficult position since our desire to encourage these feelings in others are typically thwarted by acts of aggression, self-injury, or withdrawal. Unfortunately, many caregivers believe that since the person is "unresponsive to positive reinforcement" punishment has to ensue. And, thus, the idea of friendship has to be left for a later time. The paradox of interdependence is that we have to pass through these difficult mo-

---

For caregivers, companionship involves feelings of
- Unconditional acceptance and valuing
- Being with and for the other
- Relatedness
- Mutual support
- Empathy and warmth
- Dialogue
- Sharing

ments of rejection in order to teach the meaning of companion-ship. If it were easy, there would be few behavior problems. Our belief in the dignity of the human condition is what sustains us in good times *and* hard times. The changes that gradually occur are mutual. Our giving is eventually reciprocated through the laces of affection that are woven in the emerging relationship.

Human interdependence is expressed in the practice of com-panionship. We are no more, nor any less, than those whom we serve. It is unfortunate that persons with behavioral difficulties have not yet learned this core dimension of human existence: the feeling of being at home. It is critical that parents, teachers, psy-chologists and all involved in giving care reflect on this assumption and help others move from a feeling of apartness toward one of union. If this is to unfold, we need to change and express new interactions.

The purpose of caregiving is not to rid people of behavioral difficulties, nor to instruct them to obey. The most important reason to help others to live, work, and play in the confluence of family and community life is to learn to live together. The first dimension in creating a spirit of companionship is to teach the meaning of being valued and to reciprocate it, not because anyone earns it, but because we are all human. However, unconditional acceptance and valuing are easier said than done. How should we feel when a child spits in our face, or curses us, or kicks a hole through the wall? Our culture teaches us to value orderliness, compliance, and self-achievement. These often overpower our view of what it means to be human, mask that natural longing for interdependence, and strangle our beliefs. Unconditional accep-tance means that the parent with the child having the temper tantrum has to feel and express love and affection in spite of growing impatience and feelings of rejection, since this is what will bring about closeness. The nurse with the gruff or nasty patient has to tolerate those traits and help the person feel friendship, instead of poking fun or becoming angered. The teacher with the child who is loud or disobedient has to create a new frame of mind and value the student, instead of becoming nervous at obstinacy or trouble-making. The psychiatric aide who is ordered to push and pull a violent person to a seclusion room needs to question such oppression and find ways to change hellish realities. Each of these interactions is difficult and tests our beliefs.

Empathy is not pity. It is a feeling of being one with the other. It is trying to understand why a child or adult is acting in a particular way and reflecting on the cumulative impact of each person's life history—years of segregation, submission, and isolation that gnaw away at the spirit. It is a spirit of sharing our common humanity and the belief that no one exists as a mere individual, but that we all exist interdependently. Patrick's anger is ours. His aggression is ours. His withdrawal is ours. Likewise, his emerging smile, gaze, and reaching out are ours. Empathy does not mean overprotection. It comes from our knowledge of the other and ourselves, our reality, our vulnerabilities, and our strengths and weaknesses. It is caring about the other's anger, frustrations, and rejection instead of whether the other is obeying or producing. We need to represent kindness, serenity, and peace. Empathy involves a recognition of the personal and social dimensions of what it means to be handicapped, mentally ill, poor, or

---

The emergence of companionship involves
- Seeking the other out
- A give-and-take of unconditional valuing
- Being engaged in projects together
- Feelings of safety and security

It is expressed in
- Smiles
- Warm looks
- Affectionate touching
- Words or sounds of friendship, comfort, and sincerity
- Moving toward the other
- Staying with the other
- Interacting together as friends

abandoned. It remains steadfast during good times and bad, at the depths of fury and the heights of joy. Nobody is only a student, a client, a resident, homeless, poor, or powerless. Empathy drives us to uncover the human condition and reveal its fullness, our fragility in the face of life's vicissitudes, our vulnerability to emotional disruption, and our need for being with others. We need to consider that we could be but one short step from homelessness ourselves.

How can one human express unconditional valuing to another, no matter what is transpiring? Dialogue is the concrete expression of unconditional valuing. It is a conversation in which we uplift the other. Yet it is not just words. It is our authenticity, bearing, gaze, smile, warmth, and our expression of oneness. It cannot be a role or a charade since phoniness is quickly seen and results in further rejection and distancing. The marginalized person senses and eventually responds to warmth. Dialogue can be quiet, it can consist of words or silence. It is not only what is said, but what is felt. It is the expression of our total communication, that is, our words, our gestures, our movements, and our inner feelings.

However, in the beginning, the individual has little or no reason to understand or feel any commonality with us, let alone respond in any bonded way. The very state of being shunted off to the edge of community life leaves the person almost emptied of that longing for union. Our dialogue may seem to fall on deaf ears and a hard heart. Yet our assumption is that there is a yearning within everyone in which feelings of companionship can eventually surface. It is as if the warmth of the dialogue thaws those hardened hearts until the blood of life itself flows once more.

The establishment of a feeling of companionship involves the emergence of mutually humanizing interactions. By necessity, these begin with the caregiver's initiative and are not mutual. Someone has to start the process. So the caregiver is the one who approaches, accepts, and gives unconditional valuing to the other. Yet, over time, these solitary acts begin to be returned. The caregiver's smile changes sullen looks and a kind touch changes frigidity and fear. Both begin to move toward and become engaged with one another.

Questioning Our Values

The formation of these feelings of companionship rests on our values and actions. Values without actions are devoid of meaning and actions without values are dangerous. We have a marked tendency to bury our basic feelings toward those in need. Caregiving has been overtaken by oppressive values. Obedience and independence have become the rallying calls of behavioral programs. Unquestioned attitudes have emerged over time, have blinded us to our own worth and dignity, and have led us to seek to overpower the weak and the dispossessed, often without even realizing it. This is seen in grotesque restraint and punishment practices, as well as in our day-to-day deeds. Our unquestioned acceptance of the human condition as machine-like leads us to impose these silent, oppressive beliefs, sometimes vengefully, on those who are voiceless. We hear comments such as, "I was treated that way when I was growing up. Why shouldn't that person be treated likewise?" These burdensome values are seen in daily behavior modification practices. School halls echo with the sterile commands of teachers: "Hands down. Look at me!" Discipline has become the end instead of a side effect of mutual respect. Institutional wards house thousands of voiceless people sitting, rocking, and pacing in the cold shadow of time-out rooms. Many sit in chairs with their arms and legs strapped by leather restraints because they are "a danger" to self and others, or group homes are built to house those from the drooling wards. Yet this move scarcely changes anything. Pacing, rocking, and sitting reign. Names are unknown. Faces signal fear. In these settings, the warmth of human embrace is substituted with leather straps or obedience-training programs. Many have left institutions only to be dumped onto the street. These homeless ones are invisible and pass their days and nights like ghosts.

Yet other caregivers offer hope and fight for justice: the parent who embraces the child who can hardly breath, the institutional worker who loosens the leather straps from the voiceless one's arms, the teacher who takes the confused child aside and offers words of consolation and encouragement, and countless numbers of others. These caregivers reject a culture of death and opt for a culture of life. The only discernible reply between these two ways of life rests in an unfolding awareness and understanding of values based on justice and solidarity.

> Elisa lives in an institution. Her life has been enveloped by schizophrenia that expresses its confusion in ongoing aggression and self-injury. She stands alone in her world, devoid of companionship. Motionless, she wears a padded suit and, on her head, a helmet with a black wire mask covering her iced-over eyes. Electrodes for electric shock are attached to her otherwise untouched skin. As the days and years have worn on, her caregivers have become so frustrated that they have accepted the common mandate to gain control over her. The logic of a culture of death is simple: If she hits her head, a helmet is placed on her; if she rips the helmet from her head, it is locked at the neck; if she smashes her face on the terrazzo floor, a mask is put on her face; if she rips her skin, she is fitted in a padded suit; if she perseveres in her destruction, she is shocked with a modern cattle prod. If nothing works, she is tied into a chair.

Control leads to violence, oppression, and emotional death. It might even work in the sense that the observable behavior disappears; but it only gives birth to hatred and increased distancing. The violent are overpowered with a seemingly bottomless war chest of armaments. But the result is sad to behold.

> Elisa stands alone and whispers despairing words: "Come, come, come!" Yet no one comes. Her lips quiver. Her hands tremor. Her eyes long for hope. Yet fear permeates the residence. Her presence tells caregivers to move back, and their faces tell her that fear is the rule of life. Her words, hands, and gaze are left thwarted. When she becomes belligerent and the electric shock leaves her

trembling, a caregiver sits her in a chair and ties her arms, legs, and chest with leather straps.

The caregivers in this kind of institution are not mean or cruel in their hearts. But, like Elisa, they have been "institutionalized" and locked in a nether world of violent beliefs. In college, they have learned the lonely power of reward and punishment. At work, they have been trained in the intricacies of restraint and control. At home, they most likely hug and kiss their children. But in Elisa's cottage, they lock her mask and press the cattle prod's plastic button. Like accountants, they stand with their clipboards and stopwatches to gather data on her compliance and noncompliance. They live in a world devastated by unquestioned beliefs. Our values, whether we recognize them or not, can translate into direct and ongoing domination.

This feeling of being at home needs to be expressed in our actions. We need to convey to Elisa that she is a full human being—in mind, body, and spirit. It does not make any difference how she is labeled or how many behavioral problems she might have. Mental retardation, mental illness, and other disabilities are secondary and have nothing to do with the individual's personhood. This perspective is quite difficult to put into practice. We are not dealing with behavior problems, but attempting to engage ourselves with fellow human beings with a range of unrevealed feelings. This encouragement has to be made evident in our minutest actions.

Next, we need to view ourselves as equals with Elisa. An almost natural tendency is to look down on those who cannot speak or fend well for themselves since our culture exalts achievement. We often assume the role of changing their behavior. However, a spirit of equality leads us to put aside ideas and perspectives based primarily on functional skills, independence, and individualism. We need to see the person with even the severest behavioral difficulties as our own brother or sister, since those most in need have the deepest, but unfilled, longing to be valued. We need to understand that the helping process is mutual, changing and transforming ourselves as much as the person served. We might think that we are the givers and the person with special needs is the perpetual receiver. Yet a critical element is helping the other to both accept and reciprocate unconditional valuing. The very process of reaching out to others brings wholeness to us.

We need to see our relationship with Elisa in the context of family and community life. The challenge is not to "control be-haviors," as it is so often stated, but to create community. We need to define our work in this broader reality. If we allow compliance to be the goal for one, then we hold it up as the purpose of all existence. If we permit punishment as valid for some, then we open its floodgate for all. Our posture springs out of another value system; that we are meant to live together and that this can only occur if we are creating community wherever we might be. Care-giving is a life-long process of coming together. It requires a commitment to the creation of companionship and its spreading throughout the community in families, classrooms, and work-places.

The Process of Establishing Companionship

Creating a feeling of companionship is the initial and primary goal of caregiving and involves:

1. Helping the person feel that our presence is:
   - Safe and secure
   - Consistently and predictably valuing
2. Helping the person feel that human engagement is:
   - A sign of coming together
   - An expression of ongoing valuing
3. Helping the person grasp the meaning of unconditional valuing:
   - How to accept and seek it
   - How to reciprocate and initiate it
   - How to share it with others

The Establishment of Companionship

Bringing about a mutually valued relationship means that we need to help Elisa and other marginalized people feel safe and secure with us. We have to be careful that our presence does not signal fear. When we approach the person with behavioral difficulties, we need to concentrate on nurturing rather than making demands. Our hands and our words should not be instruments of terror, but signs of valuing. Feelings of safety and security converge with the growing recognition that being with and participating side by side with others is inherently good. Participation can lead to skill acquisition and productive work, but it is much more basic. It means the growing acceptance and understanding of the significance of being with others. The acceptance of human presence and engagement with others are the cornerstones of companionship. Buildings become homes; classrooms become the garden for planting the seedlings of community; workplaces become environments for the expression of personal talent and union. Learning the meaning of human presence, engagement, and valuing leads to mutual and reciprocal feelings and interactions that signal respect and sharing. It is the fruit of the evolving fulfillment of our quest for being at home in the world. Our presence has to equate with a feeling of interdependence. Instead of yelling at a person or forcing someone to comply, our interactions need to demonstrate that we support the person and that we represent sources of companionship, not power.

Yet this spirit stands shakily when we are confronted with aggression, self-injury, or disobedience. We need to have enough strength to turn our values into meaningful interactions. But how can we remain steadfast when spit is running down our face and anger is surging at such an insult? How can we tolerate Elisa's screams and kicks when she does not want to accompany us? How can the parent open her heart when her child has a tantrum? What do feelings of companionship mean when someone is pulling out our hair? What about the homeless person who damns us and all that we do? Many caregivers say, "Well, they have to be taught a lesson! How is someone going to learn to obey, unless they suffer the consequences of their misdeeds?" Our caregiving purposes are different from those that seek obedience or control. It is at the very worst moments of aggression, self-injury, or rejection when our beliefs are the most acutely tested and when we have to remain firm in striving for companionship through our presence, engagement, and valuing.

If we were to ask what Elisa needs, some would say control, others companionship. The choice is ours. Scared, a caregiver unties Elisa's arms and legs from the wooden restraint chair where she spends most of her time. Elisa screams and thrashes since she "needs" the straps' cold embrace after so many years of such treatment; plus, she must feel that some form of meaningless demand is going to be imposed on her. The caregiver thinks, "My God, she's going to come after me with both fists flying!"; yet, she reminds herself that she needs to convey unconditional valuing. Elisa is filled with anger, not at the caregiver, but at the absurd reality in which she is warehoused. She rebels against her life condition and the assumption that any engagement with others will be oppressive. The first to free her is almost assured of attempts at aggression. Her fear meets the caregiver's anxiety, but her nonviolent courage encounters Elisa's anger. All the while, the caregiver is speaking soothing words of friendship. Elisa does not seem to have any feeling for the encouragement and affection. But the caregiver perseveres and invites Elisa to walk with her. She refuses. The caregiver still perseveres. Every move she makes expresses valuing. She knows that she has to remain nurturing in spite of Elisa's refusal. As these minutes become hours, Elisa begins to feel at ease. Every now and then she approaches the caregiver as if testing whether or not there is meaning in this new reality. She sits and then runs away. She starts doing an activity with the caregiver and then jumps up and screams. But the moments of calm and togetherness increase. Thus begins the transmission of a culture of life expressed in a slowly growing spirit of companionship.

If we step back for a moment and think about how companionship develops, it might be easier to see both its meaning and necessity for Elisa. Many lessons can be learned from normal emotional development. At the start, a mother is nurturing and unconditionally gives of herself—her time, energy, and love—to a fellow human who is totally dependent. The baby cries; she listens to those wordless expressions and knows what to do: console, help, smile, hug. All is given. The baby learns to reach out, give, smile, coo. Mutual change emerges in this unfolding bond. As dependent as the infant is, the mother, nevertheless, changes as much as the baby. She learns to give; the baby learns to receive and return valuing and eventually to spontaneously initiate it. Without this spirit, the mother would have no option but to demand obedience from the baby. Consequently, the baby would rebel, the mother would overpower the baby with shouts or spankings, and the baby would succumb to force. Unfortunately, such actions sometimes occur, and we call it child abuse. The option is for the mother to care for and care about the infant with uncalculated affection. She recognizes that the baby's well-being depends upon her giving, her warmth and affection, and her elicitation of similar feelings of union from the child. It is at this point that other developmental events begin to occur in the relationship. Expectations and responsibility increase. But the center of the relationship has been built on unconditional love. This nurturing spirit remains the guiding force in the relationship.

Among older children and adults, especially those who cling to the edge of family and community life, the bonding process with significant others is of the highest importance and needs to be consciously sought and supported among parents, siblings, peers, teachers, and other caregivers. As the child grows into adolescence and adulthood, it is expressed in friendship and companionship. A network of relationships evolves and is like a harbor that beckons the individual in distress and shelters the person from the vicissitudes of life.

We can extract some vital lessons from Elisa's reactions as they relate to the formation of feelings of companionship and what we have to pass through while still conveying unconditional valuing. She stands in fear of us, not because of deliberate cruelty, but because she lives in a culture of violence that predictably reflects relationships based on control. She finds no joy in being with any caregiver and joining in any activity, not because what she is asked to do is boring or frustrating, but because she finds no meaning in being with others. She knows that our words and gestures only bring neutrality, coldness, or pain. Our presence is like spit. Her lonely soul is filled with fear. Her feeling of repugnancy is conveyed in her distancing interactions. The more she becomes alienated, the more we typically escalate our drive for control. Yet, if companionship is to emerge in her life, we are challenged to turn fear into serenity, violence into valuing, and feelings of control into affection. We need to be ready to receive frequent rejection and hostility in our initial attempts, and we have to persevere in establishing the feeling that we represent safety and security, that we are good to be with, and that our words, presence, gestures, and other warm contacts equate with what it means to be human. Our first challenge is to reflect the fullness of her human dignity by conveying unconditional giving.

Safety and security. A profound meaning rests in our very presence. Our hands and words yield much meaning to marginalized persons. They are like instruments that either symbolize warmth and affection or oppression and control. When we raise our hand to help, this movement might generate fear, not because we consciously intend it, but because the person lives in a culture in which our hand is just one more among many violent ones. Our words of affection are just so many more syllables in a litany of orders and denigrations. These words and movements converge into a perception of what our presence so often means: fear. One of the most essential initial challenges confronting us is to teach the person that our presence, in spite of a world of control and domination, represents safety and security. When we speak it is to dialogue. When we reach out, it is to warmly help or give value. As caregivers, we have to remember that our very presence conveys strong messages. Before we utter a word or open our hands, the alienated person beings to feel who we are and what we represent.

Imagine that you are a lonely and scared child in school. The teacher approaches. What does it mean to feel in danger?

> Mary is sitting at school and the teacher coldly says, "Do your puzzle now, Mary!" The teacher has not said much of anything to the child all day except give her orders. The child sees the teacher as a stern authority figure—"Do this. Do that!" Mary becomes more frightened of her, not because the teacher is deliberately cruel, but because she sees in her little more than demanding words.

This might sound ridiculous. Is it possible that a simple thing like telling a child to do something will teach the child to have fear? The answer is "yes" if this happens day after day, year after year in a world in which the child is valued only for deeds done. Plus, it is not just spoken words, but also the tone, the superiority, and the coldness. The teacher becomes a commandant instead of a friend. There is deterioration of the human spirit over time. Our interactions are like drops of water falling on a rock. One or two drops do not make much difference. But constant drops, time after time, year after year, take their toll. Our words and acts become symbols of oppression.

Harsh words often turn into "grabbing" when the person does not do whatever it might be that they are supposed to do. Our words are like our hands, they can be instruments of valuing or domination. Caregiving is filled with euphemisms that mask violence: "physical help" is often a charade for force, "escorting" often equates with pushing and pulling another person like a bag of garbage, and "compliance" often means "Do this, or else!" The person quickly learns to fear us or rebel against us. We begin to represent feelings of danger and insecurity that distance us from the person. The gap widens.

> When Mary does not start to do her task after having been told several times, the teacher gives her a "physical prompt," taking her by the hand and moving her through the motions of compliance. This results in an emotional and physical tug-of-war with both becoming more resistant. Mary sees the caregiver approach and

Safety and security are characterized by
  • The warmth of our words, gestures, and touch
  • The serenity of our approach even when fearful
  • Our tolerance in the face of rejection
  • Our unconditional valuing in spite of noncompliance, aggression, or disruption
  • Our patience and creativity when all seems lost
  • Our rejection of dominative interactions

her heart cringes. This fear soon translates into aggression or withdrawal.

If we want to teach feelings of safety and security, we need to question what we are doing and how we are doing it. The key is to look at ourselves and ask, "What do we represent to the person: valuing or domination?" If we see the person as our equal and if we define our relationship as one of brotherhood and sisterhood, then the answer becomes more obvious. We commit ourselves to making certain that our presence signifies feelings of safety and security. Yet we need to deal with the irony of representing these feelings while face to face with rejection, disruption, or even violence.

Our interactions have to signal warmth, serenity, and tolerance. From the first instance, we need to make certain that the person interprets our presence as representing nonviolence. Warmth emanates from a strong desire to be one with the other. We have to put in check many customary reactions: demands, harshness, and objectivity. Caregiving is a very personal process that needs to summon forth feelings of friendship. At first, we should not expect acceptance since all of the person's history says control is the rule. But in time the person will begin to see us as representing safety and security.

Human engagement. Along with safety and security, it is critical to establish a sense of human engagement. As the person draws near, we need to enable the feeling that being with us and mutually participating brings us closer together, opens up on-going opportunities for sharing, and sets a backdrop for dialogue. Caregivers who are bent on bringing about behavioral control often push to have the marginalized person acquire skills based on a rationale that human value is only found in the ability to be independent. A central question is not what we can do, but who we are. Our assumption is that our life takes on meaning based on our relatedness with others. The development of our particular talents is important, but secondary if human engagement is absent. Self-reliance leaves already alienated people more isolated in a dog-eat-dog world. Our option is to teach the meaning of human engagement, that it is good to be with and participate with us and others. Doubtlessly, each of us should have the opportunity, and whatever help necessary, to develop our skills. But the affirmation of a feeling of relatedness with others is a necessary emotional precursor to skill acquisition. Just as our presence can signal fear or security, so can doing things together equate with equal repulsion, confusion, or rejection. Change occurs slowly. When a child or adult remains with us for a moment, this signals that fear is diminishing and engagement is taking root. Yet, in a split second, the individual runs away. We try to make being with us interesting, but interest is not held. The central factor in human engagement is the person's evolving desire to be with us, not his or her interest in a task. It is not some magical process by which we find an interesting task for the person to do, but in discovering his or her perception of who we are and what we represent.

To be engaged is to feel that it is good to be with the other, interact, share, and give and receive human valuing. Being together and being engaged in the flow of ordinary life communicates feelings of union. Engagement is not a relationship based on manipulation or control, but the affirmation of the other through mutual participation. For those who are marginalized, it is a critical dimension in the elaboration of companionship since it creates a common ground for being together. Yet alienated individuals have no reason to be with us. So a basic caregiving role is to bring about engagement. This is facilitated by doing activities with the person and using such a structure to express unconditional valuing.

> The teacher decides to convey a spirit of friendship to frightened Mary. Instead of ordering her to do her task, she sits beside her, reaches her hand out, and offers words of valuing while also putting the puzzle together with her. She does not mind that Mary is not "complying," but is focused on having the child feel that it is good to be near her and know that she will help her. Mary's fear begins to diminish as she learns that her teacher recognizes her value and understands her human condition. She slowly begins to participate.

In the beginning, we have to enable the elaboration of participation. Putting aside the drive to demand compliance, we have to be present with the individual and avoid domineering commands. When the person refuses to participate, the focus cannot be on "Do this, or else!"As in teaching safety and security, we need to concentrate our efforts on valuing, moving toward the person without conveying fright, and being with the other, whether or not the person does a particular activity or not.

Human engagement is characterized by
- The emerging recognition and expression of affection toward significant others
- The increasing physical and emotional approximation of the distancing person toward others
- The increasing participation in tasks and activities—doing things together
- The caregiver giving whatever help, protection, and support the person might need
- The person accepting help from others and increasingly developing and expressing personal talents in union with others
- Reaching out to others beyond the relationship with the caregiver and sharing with others
- Accepting and reciprocating human valuing

As caregivers, we have two basic choices when it comes to enabling human engagement. One is to try to make the person comply by giving rewards for good deeds and punishment for noncompliance, or to start to represent a new relationship by valuing the person and teaching the person to reciprocate this because it is good to be with us. Instead of centering our interactions on "Do this!" we need to recognize that teaching the person to be one with us is a crucial dimension of companionship. This requires us to put aside the urge to concentrate our efforts on the acquisition of skills or obedience. Rather, one of our initial roles should be to help the person participate with us, regardless of ability. The question here is not "I know Mary can do this, so she must." Instead it is "Even though she could do this, how can I help her accept being with me and secondarily do that which she has the potential to do?" We try to bring about engagement in activities, but it is more basic to find ways to have the other just be with us. As a secondary benefit, we might end up doing and completing an activity. The person, however, might be a passive participant for a time. The important thing is to draw the person toward us. Activities are vehicles for signifying that our presence and mutual participation equate with being valued.

The most common practice used in human service systems is to apply a system of reward and punishment to those who do not comply with preordained norms. This might work. If we can find the most powerful reward or punishment, many people will start to do whatever it is that we want. However, others will rebel against this. More importantly, our relationship will be built on power over the person instead of equality. So, for Mary, the teacher might give her a bottle of soda pop every time she does some task or obeys for several hours. Likewise, the teacher might take this reward away when the child fails to do the task or activity. An irony is that the caregiver becomes as imprisoned as the child in this world of the carrot and stick. The teacher is controlled by unquestioned and mechanistic practices; the child is dominated by being a mere recipient of contingent reward or punishment. This focus is on the delivery or withdrawal of privileges instead of unconditional valuing. An ongoing struggle is to drop the urge for control and establish the feeling of being together.

Unconditional valuing. The driving force behind the newly emerging meaning of our presence with others and engagement with them is our unconditional valuing. To value another is to uplift, honor, respect, listen, and reflect and share feelings, whether with words or nonverbal expressions. To do this unconditionally is to express it regardless of deeds done. It is common for a person who has been exploited and rejected, or who is simply vulnerable to emotional devastation due to handicapping or marginalizing conditions, to shun our valuing. Most individuals are accustomed to the experience of being rewarded only for deeds well done. And, since they do few things that meet the criterion for reward within this culture, they not only have little opportunity to "earn" it, but also find little meaning in it because it is most often unauthentic and mechanistic. Or, since they have been pushed and pulled so much to perform "good" behaviors, they rebel against our very presence, let alone doing something with us. The unfolding of the feeling of being valued and valuing others is the central dimension in the establishment of feelings and companionship. It can only be taught through our giving and eliciting it frequently and unconditionally. Like the other aspects of our relationship, we are confronted with its initial meaninglessness, not only in the eyes of the other, but sometimes in our own. It is impossible to give genuine value if we do not feel it ourselves and it is difficult to express it when it falls on seemingly deaf ears. Yet the act of giving it and giving it frequently, regardless of what the person might be doing or not doing, is our central task. This

---

Valuing is characterized by
- Our unconditionally giving it
- Seeking its reciprocation
- Expressing it through dialogue
- Nurturing and genuine engagement

---

process deepens its meaning for us and shares its power with the marginalized person.

> When Mary refuses to participate or throws something to the floor, the teacher does not reprimand her. She approaches her as a friend. She sits down with the child and does the particular task with her, even if she has to do everything. All the while, the teacher dialogues with the child, gives value, and gradually creates a feeling of safety and security. The child's cries lessen; the teacher feels more affectionate. She slips a puzzle piece in the girl's hand and helps her. The child gazes and smiles at the teacher.

Someone might say, "Well, I interact a lot and give positive reinforcement, but she still does not comply, and she still won't do anything. In fact, whenever I ask her to do something, she starts to throw the material on the floor, scream, or hit herself." The problem does not lie in positive reinforcement, because such reward has to be earned and Mary earns little. We are not behavioral accountants dispensing loans. Valuing someone does not depend on contingencies. It is given because she is a human being with a hunger and longing for warmth and affection. Because she is vulnerable to feelings of insecurity and fear, we need to teach her that we are continuous and certain sources of valuing. She needs to feel that it is good to be with us, that our words, our physical contact, our whole being, and all our interactions begin with, center on, and bring about human valuing.

CONCLUSION

Human interdependence starts with our beliefs. We assume that all people are mind, body, and spirit. This requires an acceptance of and dealing with much more than observable behaviors. We assume that a longing for human valuing resides in all of us. We need to recognize this in ourselves and uncover it in those who are marginalized. Furthermore, we assume that all change is mutual and that the unfolding of feelings of companionship is the ongoing purpose of caregiving. We are not only helping others but ourselves as well. To bring this new reality to fruition, we need to put three basic elements into practice: the establishment of feelings of safety and security, the goodness of human engagement, and the central role of unconditional valuing. These are the seedlings of this ongoing mutual change process.

Chapter 2
UNCONDITIONAL VALUING

Our challenge is to enable ourselves and others to enter a culture of life, a process that increasingly brings meaning to the human condition, instills hope, and establishes a process toward companionship. Unconditional valuing is the central dimension in this. Our essential role is to express to each person his or her dignity and worth by entering into a relationship based on dialogue. These interactions symbolize solidarity and prize the person through genuine and authentic expressions during good moments and difficult ones. They uplift and honor the person, not for what the individual does, but for who the individual is. We not only care for human needs, but we also care about the person because we see our own human condition in their alienation and in their longing for justice and companionship. As we try to fulfill this longing, we are creating a culture of life through our actions, interactions, and expressed beliefs. And in this, we help usher in feelings of relatedness, solidarity, and being with others.

The Central Task of Caregiving

When our interactions revolve around unconditional valuing, then our feelings and actions also reflect a full acceptance of the person, tolerance toward violent or recalcitrant acts, and empathy for the life condition of the individual. But this is no easy task. It requires a sharp consciousness that our most subtle, and seemingly irrelevant, interactions have a tremendous impact on the

> **The Central Task of Caregiving**
>
> All our interactions begin with, center on, and lead to uncondi-
> tional valuing and its reciprocation.

person's ability to accept us. A single neutral gaze, a demanding
word, or a cold touch can shout out to the already suspicious
person that we are nothing more than oppressors, even when our
intention is to value. Our interactions need to start with valuing,
including the manner in which we physically and emotionally
approach, look at, reach out to, and speak to the person. Every
move, step, and expression has to summon up a strong feeling of
genuine warmth and exude unconditional valuing. They need to
center on it. Nothing is more important than giving value. Whatever else happens, this focus has to transcend everything else. For
those trained in behaviorism, this does not mean delivering a
litany of contingent phrases; rather, it signifies a dialogue that is
ongoing, unrelated to what behaviors might be happening, and an
expression of our solidarity with the person. The most common
way to bring this about is to engage the person in an activity, not
for the sake of the activity, but to give him or her something
concrete to do while expressing unconditional valuing. This structure requires us to put aside the compulsion to teach skills or gain
compliance. Without such a structure, many caregivers flounder
after a few moments in the sea of rejection that surrounds them.
It is important to avoid conveying messages that relate to an
activity *needing* to be done; instead, the communication is, "It is
good to be with you! I will honor you regardless of what you are
doing, and I will help you learn to feel safe and valued."

Within this process, we also need to seek valuing from the
person. Besides giving it, we have to seek its reciprocation. If not,
we leave the person in a dependent position. Our posture can
become overprotection that appears kind but eventually subju-
gates and suffocates the other. It might be considered as charitable
in the sense that it "helps" the other, but it is unjust since it is not

founded on equality. Justice is based on the fulfillment of basic human rights and places us in a mutual change process with the dispossessed, with each seeking meaning in companionship. The elicitation of valuing is a process that needs to be woven into value-giving through nonforceful attempts that indicate it is fulfilling to give and receive. As we elicit and receive it, we also generate encouragement to persevere in our efforts since the slightest signs of companionship multiply our own feelings of mutuality and instill hope in us as well as in the other. We need to seek this reciprocation slowly, yet perseveringly, since so many marginalized persons fear our touch, words, or gestures. We might just seek a smile or a gaze. If the smile does not appear, we need to ask again and include these requests in our dialogue. As we give the person a few moments to consider whether to respond or not, we also continue the participation and value-giving. In due course, the person begins to learn to link our presence with being valued and valuing us.

How can we center all our interactions on valuing the other, especially when rejection is typical and even expected? We need to make a deliberate option to work among the most marginalized and accept the purpose of this engagement as unfolding our own liberation along with and because of those whom we serve. This decision enables us to confront and tolerate rejection. This commitment leads us to persevere in spite of flurries of aggression, the attempts at self-injury, and the near hopelessness of withdrawal. How can we express unconditional valuing? It is necessary to be with the person even when the individual is running from or attacking us. We have to accompany the individual and not expect immediate engagement. Remember, for the other person, everything in the relationship is likely to be meaningless at the beginning. Our words, touch, and other expressions at best signal fear or, at worst, an attack that communicates the person's anger and mistrust. Our valuing needs to rise above fear and violence. It prevents it, takes it meaning away, and replaces it with eventual feelings of union.

The Role of Technology

We need to express valuing without reservation. We have to put aside practices such as, "He needs to learn a lesson!" "Natural consequences are necessary!" and "If I value him when he's acting out, I will be reinforcing his inappropriate behavior." Such statements are a reflection of a technology based on a culture that seeks to control and results in machine-like people. Some might say, "Well, I am a behaviorist and my technology is necessary. Otherwise, I can never gain control over these behaviors." Without a doubt, techniques are important tools, but their usefulness rests in our hands and values. They need to be congruent and consistent with our beliefs. The analysis of observable behaviors can provide some knowledge relative to a person's condition, but it is only partial truth. The dual system of reward and punishment surely works to modify some behaviors, but it only partially touches the human condition. The techniques of behavior control, whether aversive or nonaversive, are based on a materialistic value-system that can cause us and others to behave like robots. We need to question the beliefs that support technology and make sure our actions are consistent with life-giving values. The establishment of the meaning of human presence, engagement, and valuing requires putting our beliefs into practice. These are complex and dependent upon much more than materials set out on a table, instructions, or daily "sessions." Their teaching necessitates and arises from our values and interactions. The role of technology in this process is important but secondary. The techniques that we muster are like the sculptor's chisel. In the hands of one person, the tool can be made to create life's images; in the hands of another, it can be an instrument of oppression.

Valuing versus Reward

Valuing is quite different from positive reinforcement. It is given, not earned. It is nurturing rather than rewarding. It occurs at good times and bad. It arises from a spirit of human solidarity, rather than from a technology used to shape specific behaviors. It is the continuous expression of our relatedness with the other. It is a dialogue of words and other interactions that affirms the sacredness of the human condition and acknowledges the common struggle in which we all find ourselves.

It is quite different from the typical carrot-and-stick approach in which good behaviors are reinforced and bad ones are punished. Even when the person is aggressive, self-injurious, or withdrawn, it leads us to center all our interactions on uplifting the wholeness of the person. All of our words, gestures, and physical interactions are intended to give value. The person screams—we continue giving value. The person swings at us in anger—we continue. The person spits in our face—we continue. The person throws material on the floor, stomps his feet, or slams the door— we continue. Of course, we also have the responsibility to prevent or diminish the force of such violence. Yet this needs to be accomplished nonviolently. At the same time, valuing needs to be associated with being with us, not in telling the person to do something, but in sitting down and doing tasks or activities. Through this we link valuing with engagement.

Life is filled with a feeling of apartness and nonparticipation. We have to find ways to engage the person in interactions with us. In the beginning, this might involve simply having the person present while we do a particular task, or it might mean that we have to move to where the person is if he or she is running from us. The key is to bring ourselves together with the person. Establishing companionship is a process that naturally involves an ebb

---

Valuing in practice is
- Given, not earned, during good moments and bad
- Centered on dialogue, that is, bringing the caregiver's life into the world of the marginalized person's through words, gestures, and physical interactions
- Involved in uplifting the person's spirit and sharing

and flow. It often requires us to do things for the person and then with them with whatever degree of support necessary. There will be moments when the person rebels. We might have to back off, but we still continue valuing.

A common caregiver reaction is, "Won't that teach the person that it is good to throw things, to hit, or to disobey?" At first this seems to make sense. We have been taught in recent years that it is wrong to reinforce maladaptive behaviors. Appropriate behaviors have to be reinforced and inappropriate ones punished or extinguished. This is one way to look at the human condition and interact with others. However, another way is to see ourselves and our purpose in a different light. In spite of the repugnancy or annoyance of the action that the other person might be involved in, we all long for feelings of being valued and being in union with others. Although it is certainly hard to see this when someone is spitting in our face, we make this assumption. We need to dig into the depths of our beliefs and see wholeness in the other. The core of this is the hunger for human interdependence. This cannot be nourished unless we fill each person's plate with valuing. Tapping into this deep wellspring is our challenge.

The power of what it means to give and receive unconditional valuing is a learning process. It cannot be given and then withdrawn. Imagine that you are starving and someone gives you food and then takes it away for whatever reason. How would you feel? The homeless person in the shelter needs comradeship, not damnation. The adult in the asylum needs intense and warm regard, not isolation. The child needs our embrace, not abuse. Valuing starts with our beliefs and is seen in our commitment to the person in the very worst moments.

Out of the blue, Ted screams "No!" several times. His size and loudness intimidate everyone. The sound echoes through the community work place. Everybody looks up. They see his large body moving. His caregiver becomes nervous, afraid, and embarrassed. Ted goes beyond yelling. He tears his shirt off, pounds his fists on the table, stands up, and hovers over the caregiver with his fists flying. The program plan says to react as "nonreinforcingly as possible" and to do a "take-down" program or a "basket-hold." The caregiver stands behind him, wraps his arms around his chest, and brings him to the floor. Another caregiver has to come over and help straddle Ted's body "until he is calm for three minutes." He is sweating, and so are the caregivers. He is scared, and so are the caregivers. He is dominated, and so are the caregivers.

Yet, we say that in this most difficult moment we need to center our interactions on valuing. Instead of overpowering Ted, there is another option: to express unconditional valuing through dialogue. This takes the best that we can give.

Later on in the day, another caregiver decides to value Ted as he begins another fury. As he stands, this caregiver stands and makes sure that his slightest movements express calming, non-violence, and nurturing. As he screams, the caregiver's warm and soothing words of value are heard. As he flails his arms, the caregiver, even with great difficulty, continues to engage him in the particular task. As he catches his breath, the caregiver places his hand in Ted's for a handshake. Ted slaps him away, but the caregiver says, "I know you are scared. I will not hurt you." At the same time, the caregiver is ready to protect himself from blows without doing violence or increasing fear. Any focus on compliance is avoided. The center of all interactions is to give him value and even to elicit it from him. Throughout forty minutes, Ted has had brief moments of calmness—catching his breath, rocking, and looking around. The caregiver has stood and sat with him. He has done a task for him and then with him. All along he has conversed with him about friendship, doing things together, and feeling safe. Ted increasingly senses the warmth of the tone and starts to scream and thrash less. Instead of hitting the caregiver's hand, he starts to let him touch his and a faint smile emerges.

If the caregiver had tried to reinforce Ted for compliance, he would have been left to flounder in his confusion. Positive reinforcement is totally different from dialogue. The first is contingent; the other is given with complete acceptance and disregard for what might have been done or not done. Positive reinforcement is generally onesided; the caregiver delivers it as a postal worker delivers a letter to an occupant—impersonal, disconnected, and irrelevant. It lacks qualities of authenticity and warmth. Unconditional valuing is ongoing, based on dialogue, and noncontingent. While recognizing that it will often hold little or no meaning in the beginning, our task is to teach Ted that our valuing quenches the thirst for being with others and quells the hunger for the unconditional affirmation of what it means to be human.

Yet domination exists in the very flesh of our culture. It is in constant conflict with solidarity. It flows in our veins, and we often allow oppression to freeze over our being. But we have the ability to question our reality and to opt for solidarity. Some make this choice; others do not. A glance around our world reveals homelessness amidst opulence, shelters where food has to be earned, schools where children are lined up as little soldiers in a constant drill, and institutions where the mentally ill, the mentally retarded, and the aged are subjected to the bleakest forms of behavior modification. In these settings, practices such as the use of seclusion, cattle prods, drugs, and restraints are a way of life, but a life that brings about feelings of apartness. The ability to opt for a culture of life lies in our hearts, minds, and actions. It is the marginalized who can transform our values and practices if we open our eyes. This option will bring life where emotional death has reigned.

We are enculturated in domination from our earliest years. We learn that it is better to be the best, to compete and step over those in our path, and to pursue self-reliance as if it were the ultimate good. Professionals come from schools that produce behavioral change experts entrenched in a materialistic view of the human condition and trained to efficiently and effectively modify behaviors. Rules and regulations are written with behaviorism and behavioral practices as basic assumptions. In-service training concentrates on physical force, in the name of self-defense, to deal with aggression and self-injury. Caregivers practice "individual planning" that removes the human spirit from the caregiving process. So our option requires ongoing questioning and renewal.

Domination is most frequently seen among caregivers bent on teaching compliance or eliminating maladaptive behaviors. These rallying calls are the harbingers of control through force and this is the parent of domination.

> Little 4-year-old Maria is giving her mother many problems. She is a pretty girl and shows much affection, but she does only what she wants to do, when she wants to do it, and only for as long as she is interested. She is running her mother ragged. Frustration is apparent on her face. Helpless, the mother goes to a local behavior management clinic and asks for help: "I need a way to deal with my daughter's tantrums." The response is swift: "Every time that Maria cries out, tell her in a firm voice, 'No!' Then order her to put her hands down for ten seconds." So the mother goes home and carries out this efficiently packaged prescription. Sometimes the child obeys; at other times she cries incessantly. The mother begins to feel like a monster as she yells the firm "No!" Their relationship is beginning to worsen, and the child is not improving. The mother feels like a boot camp instructor more than a nurturing mother. Even though she had been frustrated and tired, she had at least felt like a mother prior to the behavioral prescription.
>
> She returns to the clinic and reports her problems. The interdisciplinary team meets, considers the child some more, and then says, "It is just a matter of time and consistency. Keep carrying out the program. It will work. You are probably not doing it right." Back home, the mother continues to yell at her child and to order her to put her hands down. After several weeks of getting nowhere, she decides to make a change. She sees that her interactions are as emotionally destructive as the child's. She feels that, even though it might be possible to simply overpower her daughter, it is much better to return to a nurturing relationship.
>
> That evening, when Maria is crying and refusing to have her hair brushed, the mother starts to sing a nursery rhyme. Instead of focusing on the crying and pushing away, she decides it is more motherly to express warmth and kindness toward her daughter. So she sings while starting to brush the child's hair. Maria looks quizzically for a moment and then sits on her mother's lap, smiles, and

gazes into her mother's eyes. This begins a return to the mother's original and natural relationship with her daughter. It will be a long and difficult process, but fulfilling for both.

What the mother had decided to do was to renounce violence and recommence centering her interactions on valuing. This nurturing is essential in the development of mutually humanizing emotions and feelings of companionship. As caregivers, we can either represent domination or valuing. We can either teach apartness or union. Domination is most frequently almost unnoticeable acts such as coldness and detachment in our words and deeds. Perhaps domination seems to be too strong a term for that cold gaze or disinterested conversation. Yet every interaction matters. It is their cumulative effect over days, months, and years. Likewise, valuing is often silent and is delicately woven in the fabric of our interactions—the way we move, our tone, and our touch. Fortunately, these fragile threads become stronger as we weave them into laces of affection.

CONCLUSION

Caregiving requires conscious decisions that reflect our values. It leads us to teach the meaning of our presence and that of the person, the goodness of human engagement, and the centrality of valuing. Yet, as we have seen, this is easier said than done. Underneath this rests a life process and a purpose that we are all struggling to make unfold. If we are to value the child or adult with severe difficulties, we need to constantly recognize that we are involved in a mutual life-giving process. If we value the other, we are valuing ourselves. We transform ourselves as much as we help the other. As caregivers, we have to see the human condition as consisting of much more than observable behaviors. This mind–body–spirit assumption places us as co-participants in a process of becoming more fully human. It liberates everyone from the loneliness and self-isolation of individualism. It makes history by freeing us to transform our lives, moving us from apartness to union. Caregiving cannot be a here-today, gone-tomorrow process. It has to endure with consistency, stability, and personalization. Companionship is not an end, but a life-long process that expands outwardly. We are called on to make a life commitment. Our central role is to bring about a spirit of unconditional valuing. This requires a movement away from dominative interactions and a commitment to the development of interactions centered on warmth and authenticity. The underlying challenge is to choose between domination and valuing. This, then, also helps the marginalized person learn union instead of apartness.

Chapter 3
OUR INTERACTIONS
Valuing versus Domination

Before worrying about others' actions and interactions, let us question what we do and how we do it. Caregiving interactions are complex and bear directly on how others interact with us. We need to reflect on ourselves before examining others. Many traits and practices make it hard for us to focus on being value-givers. If we want to start centering our interactions on valuing, we need to look at all our interactions and question what they are expressing. Our challenge is to dramatically increase those that symbolize valuing and decrease those that represent any feeling of overpowering the person. The purpose of this is to establish the beginning of a new relationship based on the desire to be with one another instead of obedience to our commands.

A Culture of Life

Companionship gives life and enrichment. It views even the most aggressive person as a whole person and is based on equality. We are no more, nor any less, than the person served, even those with the severest behavioral difficulties. It generates newness and is expressed in an authentic desire to be one with the person. We assume the commitment to start it since the person served does not yet know its meaning and reality. It is marked by genuine warmth,

tolerance, and respect. It includes our beliefs and actions, relationships, and dedication to an ongoing struggle. It is based on our
acceptance of the interdependence of all people, powerful and
powerless, fast and slow, productive and nonproductive. Companionship is our central purpose in a culture of life. Unconditional
valuing is our primary process, and dialogue is our fundamental
instrument for its expression.

Caregiving is historic since it helps us and others change life
direction and enter into a spirit of full personhood and solidarity.
It frees us from the machine-like approaches that we are trained
to do in individualized cookbook plans and functional analysis and
problem solving. It enables us to become more human through
the deepening of our warmth, tolerance, and affection. It brings
about feelings of oneness and relatedness. This requires us to
uncover and reveal these feelings and share them with the other.
A culture of life embraces the longing for companionship as the
center of the human condition, but it does not stop there. It
nurtures the development of community life and the coming together of all marginalized people—the poor, the exploited, and
the institutionalized. We are in the midst of a struggle. As caregivers, we can be a people of life or death, hope or sorrow, and
valuing or domination. If we enter the caregiving relationship as
value-givers, and remain steadfast, we will help fulfill feelings of
companionship in ourselves and in others.

The overall challenge is to be a creator of a culture of life
through the struggle to reach out toward those who are marginalized. In practice, this means that parents take the time and
energy to value their children, teach them to share with others,
and center their interactions on a pattern of valuing. Of course,
there will be moments when patience is raw or when other problems and circumstances make it next to impossible to do this.
However, the issue is the direction in which the parent is taking
the child, and this requires a commitment that transcends intolerance. The same applies to our interactions with all other
marginalized people. A culture of life means that we put aside
punishment practices in favor of justice. We do away with compul-

Psychological Postures	
Culture of life	*Culture of death*
Life-giving	Destructive
Mutual	Obedience-centered
Wholeness-centered	Stimulus-response based
Democratic	Authoritarian
Generative	Oppressive
Authentic	Manipulative
Freeing	Subjugating
Participatory	Self-centered
Unconditional	Contingent
Interdependent	Independent
Solidarity-based	Self-reliant

sions to impose compliance in favor of mutual engagement. We lessen the primacy of independence and elevate human interdependence. We begin to see the gnawing away kinds of interactions that drive vulnerable individuals from us, and we seek to change any signs of overpowering.

A culture of life cannot be left to mere rhetoric; it has to be made concrete. It is the parent hugging the child instead of spanking. It is the teacher consoling the frightened child instead of yelling. It is the psychiatrist taking the time to listen to the parent or patient, not just handing out a tranquilizer. It is the social worker who does not give up and fights for human rights. It is the street worker who helps to organize the homeless to demand jobs and housing, not just soup and blankets. A culture of life is immediately felt in warm and family-like interactions, shared meals, mutual activities, and valuing interactions. It is seen in the manner of school children, the strong learning to help the weak and the active learning to reach out to those who are isolated. Caregiving is a moral and political act that leads us to imagine the possibility of justice through changing individual and social realities. It moves us to look at the systems in which we oppress people and transform violent practices.

Perhaps a culture of death sounds too strong to describe the life conditions of marginalized people and the acts that we perform. It might make more sense if we conjure up images of the poor and dispossessed on death rows, or the grotesque punishment practices that occasionally make the news such as the use of cattle prods, white sound helmets, and spankings. But a culture of death is any life pattern that equates with any form of domination, any expression of superiority, and any focus on the "self." It is emotionally destructive, but slowly eroding the spirit rather than quickly consuming it. It views people as robot-like, with each having the duty to adapt to preordained rules and expectations. Behavior modification is a perfect technology for a culture of death since it is based on control and our self-assumed authority to change those individuals who do not fit into the world of normalcy. And it asks for no substantial change from us, only technical competency.

A culture of life recognizes that caregiving is a life project that makes no distinction between our value as humans and that of the most rebellious homeless person, the most recalcitrant and obnoxious child, or the slowest person with mental retardation. It leads us to interact as brothers and sisters and as absolute equals. Yet it also asks us to assume the commitment to initiate the establishment of a spirit of companionship. It inspires us to struggle against daily oppression and organize others to assure justice. An option for a culture of life is an integrative, interactional, and liberating process. It is integrative in that it calls for an acceptance of the whole person, not just external behaviors. It is interactional in that is recognizes the commonality of basic human needs and the mutuality of the struggle to fulfill them. It is liberating in that it helps each to come together and become more.

CAREGIVING POSTURES

Caregiving practices reflect four distinct interactional postures. Overprotection is a common posture that arises out of a charitable view of marginalized people. It involves a value system that holds that our role is to help the misfortunate, care for them, and keep them subservient. It is often seen as warm and kind. However, in the long run, it smothers the individual. It emanates from an attitude of doing good, but it does not include any personal change and ignores the surrounding political and economic realities that cause and multiply marginalization. It ignores oppression and exalts one-sided helping.

A more common interactional posture, authoritarianism, is expressed by those who take an authoritarian posture. It is from this posture that industrialized nations pound in the belief that self-reliance is the essential good of the human condition. This posture is perfectly congruent with behavior modification since it is based on external control and the pursuit of compliance through reward and punishment. Authoritarian acts place us in a lofty and unassailable position over others. A related posture is frigidity. The third posture reflects the view that humans are nothing more than machine-like creatures who only respond to external stimuli. Caregivers who neither have, nor desire, any relationship with the individual served possess this view. Their words and touch are mechanistic because they pride themselves on objectivity, efficiency, and data collection. They do not see themselves or others as being human; they deliver reward and punishment to faceless occupants. This posture, and its twin, authoritarianism, is the ideal expression of orderliness and efficiency, yet it is devoid of spirit and is sterile.

A fourth value system that leads to distinct caregiving practices is based on human solidarity, in which we recognize frailty and struggle, oppression and injustice, and needs and longings. It conveys a feeling of union through unconditional valuing, tolerance toward rebellious interactions, and the expression of affection in the face of hatred and anger. It is the force that mobilizes caregivers to change oppressive situations and enables the marginalized to recognize oppression and fight for justice. Solidarity means equality: No parent has any more worth than the child, no teacher is above the student, no psychiatrist or psychologist is any more than the patient. The only difference is that our initial role is to assume the responsibility for mutual change. The parent has the unique obligation to nurture and guide the child. The teacher has the responsibility to unfold the child's talents. Each profession assumes responsibility for specific dimensions of the human condition. Indeed, through the act of caregiving, the marginalized awaken us to injustice and teach us to forget ourselves and reach out toward others.

ESTABLISHING COMPANIONSHIP

When we walk through a typical "program" for children, the homeless, those with mental retardation, the mentally ill, the aged, or any other marginalized group, what do we so often see? Loneliness and isolation often reign. Feelings of condescending friendliness are reserved for "recreation" programs, special social events, and assembly line learning or working. Silence prevails and heads are bowed in compliance. Yet in other settings smiles can be seen, affectionate sounds can be heard, and solidarity can be felt. The difference is in the spirit brought and instilled by caregivers.

Mutuality emerges in the caregiving relationship based on the perception that we are a life companion with the other. This is a phenomenon in which mutual valuing transcends all other questions. However, we have to initiate and carry the weight of this process in the beginning without being overly anxious for any reciprocation. The first hours, days, or weeks are akin to preparing the soil for a harvest. We should not expect to walk in and have trust. No, the first days involve tilling the soil, nurturing it, and awaiting the inevitable harvest. The first dimension of the establishment of companionship places the entire challenge on us. What the soil needs is unconditional acceptance and valuing, warm hands reaching out to cold hearts, and protection without smothering. It is a matter of doing away with our domineering attitudes and actions and opting for unconditional valuing, deep and broad enough to make deserts fertile. And because it is just

and mutual, it means that we also have to draw valuing and participation out of the person, not just to equalize the relationship,
but also because the poor can give more than the rich, the slow can
quicken the fast, and those on the periphery have a deeper view
than those in the middle.

The Elements of Companionship

Our research has led us to try to uncover the basic factors that
help lead to companionship, that is, the interactions that we engage in that strongly communicate our desire and commitment to
value the other person at any time, in any circumstance, and,
thereby, bring us into a process of becoming a companion. After
examining our experiences with hundreds of children and adults
with severe behavioral difficulties, we found that unconditional
valuing is the most critical factor that influences the establishment
of companionship and the significant lessening of behavioral
difficulties. Other important factors are warmly helping others,
seeking valuing from them, and protecting them whenever they
seek to hurt themselves or others. We also found several variables
that express domination and work against a culture of life: the
contingent use of reward and punishment, demanding assistance,
and the use of restraint. Value-centered expressions and the
elimination of their domineering counterparts were found to be
the most significant variables in the establishment of feelings of
companionship. We also discovered that, often unknowingly, most
caregivers display subtle, but intense, forms of domination and
that it is necessary to become aware of and change these as we
concentrate on the expression of valuing. The subtlety of both
valuing and domination can be seen in the simplest interactions—
the way we look at someone, touch them, speak to them, and how
we present ourselves physically, verbally, or gesturally. It is the
constellation of these interactions that has to be considered and
dealt with before and during our involvement with marginalized
people.

Increasing Our Value-Centered Interactions	
• Value-giving	• Value-elicitation
• Warmly helping	• Protection

VALUE-CENTERED DIMENSION

The cluster of caregiver interactions that relates to valuing the other is our first concern. These value-centered interactions are in direct competition with our tendency to dominate. We need to dramatically increase these before concerning ourselves with the behavioral problems of others.

Value-Giving

Value-giving refers to any action on the part of the caregiver that recognizes and expresses the dignity, worth, presence, and participation of the person. It conveys genuineness, sincerity, and honesty. It represents solidarity with the person. It is given through words, touches, gestures, or any other form of verbal or nonverbal expression. Indeed, most often what we "say" is expressed without words—by the tone of our voice, the softness of our gaze, and the serenity of our movements. They are interactions that prize the other with genuine and warm regard. They are honest, direct, and sincere, not mere role playing. They are given at any time, not just contingently. In fact, most frequently, valuing is given regardless of any particular behavior. It is given for who the person is, not for what the individual does. It requires a deep commitment on our part to perceive the wholeness of the other, a commitment that propels us to give respect and friendship regardless of what might be transpiring. Its expression emanates from our whole being. It can be seen in our physical, verbal, and gestural interactions.

Physical valuing refers to any interactions involving physical contact that expresses honor and respect, such as patting the shoulder, handshakes, hugs, or any other forms of value-based contact.

Verbal valuing refers to any interactions involving words or vocalizations that express these feelings, as heard in authentic and joyful vocal expressions. Sometimes these are playful, and at other times serious, but they always uplift the fullness of the person.

Gestural valuing is indicated in interactions such as smiles, nods of approval, and any other gesticulations that express the person's worth as an equal being.

Value-giving tells the person that we represent safety and security. It conveys the recognition that our interactions express warm and genuine feelings of oneness. These are more than mere rewards because positive reinforcement is only given for deeds done according to preordained norms. These interactions are given rather than earned. They are expressed in even the most difficult moments and are more than just praise. They are an ongoing dialogue with the person that demonstrates, through words, gestures, and touch, the acceptance of the other in spite of ongoing rejection. These interactions are central to what we do as caregivers.

Elizabeth has broken off with reality. She closes her eyes and only sees the dead. She recites the names of her 70 years of losses. Each name rolls from her lips and falls on deaf ears. She bows, bends over, and picks up an imaginary chalice. One caregiver scornfully laughs, but another decides to value her. This woman approaches Elizabeth and tells her, "You are seeing all those whom you have lost. They are piled high, each one recalling hope lost." Holding Elizabeth's trembling hands, the caregiver expresses warmth and serenity. Who knows what Elizabeth is thinking? In a few moments her rapid litany of the dead slows and she glances at the caregiver, whose kind valuing continues, respecting Elizabeth's disconnected flow of thought, gently breaking in with a dialogue about loss and hope and eliciting feelings of comfort. She asks her to reach out while accepting her driven language. She makes sure that her words and gestures are sisterly and that her touch is loving. Everything she does expresses valuing in spite of Elizabeth's disconnected words. She does not assume that Elizabeth's reactions will involve immediate acceptance, nor even that she will understand her giving. But she does suppose that within Elizabeth lurks a longing for relatedness and that, in due course, she will feel the warmth of value-giving and return from her exile in the land of the dead.

A marked difference exists in the way we typically value someone. Caregivers have been trained to be contingent, only "delivering reward" after someone has done a specific behavior that is regarded as "rewardable." Yet Elizabeth was doing nothing to merit reward. Even if given, contingent reward would have been transparently artificial since it would have been perceived as a script in a bad play in which the caregiver was an actress instead of a companion. Reward would have been filled with phoniness. More importantly, its contingent nature would have dictated that Elizabeth would have received precious little attention since she was totally disconnected from reality. If caregivers wait to praise the child or adult only for deeds well done, these individuals will be waiting a long time. And since reward will not work, caregivers have to dig into their tool box of punishment practices. For these reasons, we distinguish between reward and unconditional valuing, which is noncontingent, sincere, authentic, ongoing, and fully empathic. This is Elizabeth's only hope and it needs to be our driving commitment.

Value-giving can take an infinite number of forms in its verbal, gestural, and physical expressions. In other words, value-giving can involve telling stories about ourselves or others, with themes related to friendship, togetherness, home, and the reality in which we live or work. In Elizabeth's instance, value-giving was expressed in the caregiver's warm caress of her hands, in her kind words, and in her smiles and warm gaze. The caregiver needs to have a moral imagination, that is, the ability to see and describe the world so as to evoke understandings and feelings congruent with personal and social justice. Elizabeth had suffered a mountain of losses and their weight had finally overcome her. So the caregiver spoke of life, hope, and purposefulness. However, our nonverbal expressions are as critical as our verbal ones, for example, the way we look at and touch the person, our tone of voice, which may convey warmth and affection, and our physical interactions, such as pats on the back. Each way in which we communicate has to reflect the fulfillment of the basic longing for companionship within a context of justice.

Reciprocity Eliciting

Even if caregivers give plenty of reward, they often leave the person in a passive and dependent state since it can be a lopsided process. The marginalized individual is viewed as the receiver and we as the givers. This places us in an unjustly powerful position and leaves the dispossessed more powerless. The center of the human condition is not only our valuing others, but their empowerment to value us. We need to avoid being "nice" and focus on simply being one with the other. It is reciprocation that draws us into equality, so we have to teach the goodness of being valued as well as value-giving. Reciprocity eliciting refers to any interaction on the part of the caregiver that has as its expressed purpose the evocation of the expression of valuing on the part of the person toward the caregiver. This is meant to encourage and teach the person to return and initiate value-giving toward others. It is as significant as any valuing that the caregiver conveys. Like value-giving, these interactions need to be elicited from the person in a spirit of companionship, avoiding force or a condescending attitude. They initially depend on our seeking them from the person.

Physical reciprocity eliciting refers to those interactions on the part of the caregiver that physically attempt to draw the return of value-giving from the person, such as placing one's hand in another person's for a handshake, assisting the person to embrace by placing his arms on one's shoulders, or assisting the person to signal delight by touching her face for a smile.

Verbal reciprocity eliciting refers to any words or sounds on the part of the caregiver that have the purpose of eliciting the same as the above, such as asking for a handshake, a hug, or a smile. These expressions generally take place in a context of camaraderie and doing things together.

Gestural reciprocity eliciting refers to any gesticulations on the part of the caregiver that have the same purposes as the above, as seen in the caregiver extending his or her hand for a handshake or a hug, indicating a smile, or looking warmly at the person.

Reciprocity eliciting is intended to draw valuing toward ourselves and then toward others. It indicates to the person that relationships are not paternalistic, nor based on authoritarian attitudes. Rather, they are founded on equality. Reciprocity eliciting involves any caregiver contacts that are designed to help the person learn to return valuing interactions. By teaching the person to both accept and give human valuing, we create a relationship common to friends instead of a client-centered one. These involve direct appeals or gestures to the person to smile, to shake hands, and other typical symbols of a bonded relationship. More significantly, they involve the creation of an ongoing dialogue with the person since they lead to the eventual expression of authenticity. In the beginning, this is more of a monologue since the person does not yet have or even know what companionship is. But with perseverance a spirit of dialogue begins to take hold.

Reciprocity eliciting encompasses all of our interactions that we can muster to draw valuing out of the person. It is often woven into our value-giving and warm helping. If we are physically helping a person, it might include saying to the person, "As we are doing this, we ought to stop for a second and give a handshake just to show that we are friends." Such a simple statement is much more than mere words. It is the way we say it, the manner in which we approach the person, and the felt warmth of our words and touch. In addition, during the act of helping, we might be simultaneously caressing the person's hand, thus increasing the valuing many times. Reciprocation also includes a precise definition of what it is, that is, we need to learn to seek the slightest signs of movement toward us. For example, a handshake might just be the person's willingness to touch our hand rather than a firm grasp, or a smile might be a furtive, but warm, glance.

> When the caregiver reaches out to Elizabeth, her intention is to teach Elizabeth to express warmth toward her in spite of her fixation on death. As the caregiver continues listening and talking, she concentrates on telling a story about friendship and sharing. Her words, touch, and facial expressions are warm, but she also makes sure that she places her hand in Elizabeth's for a handshake and touches her face for a smile. Of course, Elizabeth initially wants to rebel against these "intrusions." But the caregiver's gentleness subdues the fear. She perseveres in the process, and finally a smile appears on Elizabeth's face and her hand opens. Words of death slow, and the caregiver is enabled to connect more with Elizabeth's feelings of life.

Helping Warmly

Giving warm help refers to any caregiving interaction done in a patient and tolerant manner to effectuate mutual participation and a shared spirit of engagement without causing any violence. It involves the process of teaching or utilizing concrete skills that enable increased opportunities for engagement and also the expression of friendship in the helping relationship. Warmly helping includes interactions to prevent disruption or to maintain or increase the person's capacity to participate. These interactions convey a spirit of mutuality, not the imposition of demands as seen in physical or emotional tugs-of-war. The warmth dimension signifies that the caregiver is assuming responsibility for empowering participation and valuing, regardless of any behavior. Warmth is conveyed in the caregiver's nurturing tone, softness of touch, and thoughtful presence. The person learns that being with and participating with the caregiver is good. Warmth can be seen in empathy, caring, respectfulness, and trust. It reflects solidarity with the person, not overprotection or bossiness. The frequent linking of engagement with unconditional valuing generates an understanding and feeling that these phenomena are of the same cloth.

Warm physical help refers to those interactions that promote participation through any physical interventions, such as working hand-in-hand with the person; prompting movements, such as tapping the person's elbow; or any other physical contact that elicits or attempts to elicit participation. It avoids any force or sense of demand.

Warm verbal help refers to those interactions whose purpose is to promote the same as the above, except words or vocalizations of any kind replace physical intervention. It is helpful to express any verbal instructions within a context of dialogue and in a spirit of "We are doing this together."

Warm gestural help refers to those interactions whose purpose is to promote the same as the above, except gestures replace words or physical contact, as seen in interactions such as pointing to the next step in a task, moving materials closer, and making signs that indicate the correct movement. It needs to be remembered that even gestures have a "tone" and their expression needs to be an invitation rather than a demand.

A teacher helps Timothy, who refuses to participate, by avoiding any direct focus on compliance. He slides to the floor; she follows. He throws a puzzle piece; she ignores it and continues to do the task with him. He does not want to pick up the next piece; she does it for him. The next time she places it softly in his hand. When she sees that he is going to throw it again, she goes ahead and places it on the puzzle board for him. As he lets her work with him, she gives him more physical help, making sure that her touch is affectionate and nonthreatening. She includes their activity in her story, making any instructions a part of it. All the while she is tolerating his screaming, kicking, and spitting. Every move she makes is intended to sincerely give and elicit valuing while helping him feel engagement is good.

Warmly helping involves a broad range of interactions. The expression of warmth is the critical dimension in this variable. It includes the expression of words that are not commands, touch that is not forceful, and gestures that are not mechanistic. For a person who has trouble doing tasks, it might mean a parent working hand-over-hand with a child, but taking extreme care to use their hands as instruments of affection. For a caregiver working among the homeless, it might mean inviting the person into the kitchen, not being a passive recipient of charity, but an active participant in justice-making—organizing the street people, running the shelters and soup kitchens, publishing a newsletter, and speaking out. For a person living with someone who is mentally disorganized, it might mean the avoidance of words, sitting down and doing the task together, and making sure that the pace of the help is congruent with the person's mood. If the person refuses to participate, the caregiver might go ahead and do the task for the person. Remember the main intent of this variable is human engagement, not skill acquisition or compliance. The caregiver has to understand that whatever the importance of the task, the more important phenomenon is to indicate through deeds that doing things together is crucial.

Helping interactions are perhaps the most frequent caregiving ones. But, these are not always warm. Indeed, they are frequently cold and mechanistic, even written out as if the caregiver is playing a role rather than forming a friendship or carrying out programmed commands rather than expressing valuing. Or they are condescending, treating the person as garbage or as a mere object. In warmly helping interactions, caregivers focus on one of the most critical variables they engage in. Since a person with behavioral difficulties has trouble participating, caregivers spend much time and energy getting them to do tasks and activities, protecting them, and preventing harm. Warm help means that in any interaction caregivers convey a feeling of the goodness of doing things together and being together. Demands are replaced by caregivers doing activities with the person; compliance is replaced by caregivers enabling participation; reward is replaced by unconditional valuing; monologue is replaced by dialogue. Warm helping also means that we have to change our perspective on skill acquisition and productivity, the be-all and end-all of many programs. The initial and ongoing central reason for helping is to eliminate feelings and actions related to apartness and move the caregiver and person toward an evolving friendship and the expression of mutual trust.

Protecting

Protecting refers to those caregiving interactions that are used to prevent actual or possible harm to the person or anyone else, whether through acts of self-injury, aggression, or property destruction. The primary factor involves the avoidance of any kind of immobilization, even for a split second. Protection includes actions such as shadowing a person's movements to prevent being hit, blocking hits, or any form of contact that occurs at a particular moment when harm is imminent. These also include actions that prevent disruptiveness. These do not include any form of restraint or forced movements. They do not include those packaged approaches that make caregivers appear as boot camp instructors. Most hospitals, institutions, and even community programs train caregivers to fight violence with violence through courses that teach the self-defense and physical restraint techniques. But protective actions do not involve such tactics. They prevent the escalation of violence, they neither immobilize nor humiliate the person, and they are brief and must be accompanied by engagement and valuing. An irony is that during the worst moments, caregivers need to be the most valuing and help with the greatest degree of warmth.

Physical protection refers to those momentary interactions that the caregiver uses to physically prevent harm while avoiding any bodily immobilization. Grabbing sends a clear message that violence and despair can only be responded to with force and disrespect. Protection includes shadowing and blocking, as well as any other form of physical contact, as long as they do not immobilize the person and are linked with simultaneous re-engagement and valuing. Shadowing involves caregivers moving their hands or arms in unison against any attempts at self-injury or aggression, but without immobilizing the other. Blocking involves caregivers using their hands or arms to stop such attempts by allowing the person to hit them in such a manner. Protection's purpose is to shelter the person or others from harm in a warm, nonviolent manner. It does not lead to overpowering. It increases the concurrent likelihood of participation and valuing. For example, when a caregiver raises his or her arm to block a hit, this is protection. Another example is the use of momentary environmental arrangements by watching where one sits or stands, enough to prevent harm and yet continue participation.

Verbal protection refers to the same as the above, except words or vocalization replace physical contact. For example, as a person's hand moves to strike, the caregiver might say, "You know, what I need is a handshake!" And at the same time the caregiver touches the person's hand and converts it into a handshake.

Gestural protection refers to the same as above, except gesticulations replace words or touch. For example, the caregiver might lift a hand and signal a playful "Hold it!" and then give more help.

In addition to valuing and warmly helping, caregivers also have the responsibility to protect themselves and others. The very nature of behavioral difficulties implies that someone can be hurt by acts of aggression or self-injury. Caregivers need to do everything possible to avoid harm while simultaneously valuing the other. Yet, it does not mean that people are restrained or punished. Protection signifies that caregivers avoid any form of immobilization. Nonviolence is a basic rule in caregiving. Aggression toward self or others should not be combated by aggression, nor anger by anger, nor rebellion by overpowering. Of course, we can mobilize enough physical strength to dominate the weak and powerless. But if valuing is to permeate our interactions, control through force is not an option. Yet, occasionally caregivers are confronted with extreme physical danger to themselves or others. A fundamental mandate is that harm should come to no one. We make a distinction between protection and restraint. The former's intention is to assure safety through nonviolence, while the latter seeks to overpower and even teach a "lesson." Protection involves a concentrated focus on the prevention of the escalation of violence, and this requires a clear desire on the part of caregivers to want to value the other person instead of gaining control. It includes caregivers watching where they sit or stand if they think violence might occur. It also requires ongoing participation even in the midst of fury and, of course, unconditional valuing. It means avoiding harm by being alert to the possibility of violence, or, if necessary, protecting ourselves, the individual, or others by blocking hits with our hands or arms. A protecting caregiver does not grab, order the person to stop, or carry out a martial arts physical intervention. Occasionally we will take a blow, scratch, or kick. When an action like this happens once, seek to prevent it thereafter. More importantly, caregivers need to increase their valuing, nurturing, and soothingness at these most difficult times.

> When Timothy kicks his teacher once, she quietly moves her legs out of his reach. When he spits in her face, she does not react to him in anger, but slides slightly out of the spit's range. When he hits her arm, she does not flinch and stop, but rather continues to participate and dialogue with him.

Some might say, "Well, he is just a small child. What do you do when the person is big and mean, really violent?" Our response is essentially the same: prevent the escalation of violence, avoid any harm by using protective actions, and watch your physical position. More importantly, the caregiver has to focus attention more deeply on valuing.

> Matthew is over six feet tall and has a mean look. He lives in a group home and spends much of the time in a locked room near the kitchen—an absurd contradiction of being at home. He has sent several staff to the hospital. Everyone fears him; no one wants to be near him or ask him to do anything. His caregivers' goals have been to teach him to comply and to eliminate his aggression. His psychiatrist has diagnosed him as antisocial. His behavioral psychologist has concluded that he has to be isolated and restrained "whenever necessary." His caregivers have been taught to make him do his daily activities whether he wants to or not "because compliance is important." Two caregivers have to work with him and forcefully take his arms and make him go through the motions of compliance. He rebels almost every time and becomes increasingly aggressive. His fists swing and lash out. However, the program plan has considered this "escalating noncompliance" by describing a "takedown" procedure in which the caregivers "physically escort" him away from others and bring him to the floor with whatever force might be necessary. He is then held until he calms down.

Restraint is common, whether it consists of physically subduing someone, placing individuals in straitjackets or other devices, or drugging them into oblivion. Thousands upon thousands of children and adults lay supine on floors with caregivers straddling their bodies, stand in the corner of seclusion rooms slamming their heads against the wall, or sit in wooden chairs with their arms and legs strapped. What is our option for Matthew? How can we protect him and ourselves while still unconditionally valuing him and warmly helping him to become engaged with us?

> Because he becomes frightened easily, another caregiver decides to approach him in a soothing and quiet manner. As the

caregiver approaches him, Matthew says, "No!" and swings his arm. The caregiver remains calm and continues to soothingly give him value. There are no demands on Matthew at this moment, but the caregiver has a task ready to do by herself with Matthew simply being nearby. She initiates a dialogue that expresses her view of him as good and kind, that it is good to be together and that she wants to be his friend. She says, "I know that you are afraid, but I will not hurt you." She makes sure that she stands a short distance out of arm's reach in case he tries to swing at her. He tests her momentarily by lifting his arm up, but she continues to do the task while keeping one eye on his movements. For a split second, he grabs her hair, but she places a piece of the task in his hand and helps him participate. She increases her valuing. His drive to become aggressive slowly subsides.

This is easier said than done because at any given moment the caregiver is not only protecting herself, but also warmly helping him, unconditionally valuing him, and eliciting value from him. Each of these factors are called for in varying mixes at different moments. The guiding rule, even during violence, is that all her interactions are value-centered. Protection is important and needs special attention since it can easily cross over the boundary to restraint. It involves the use of our words, gestures, or physical interactions, but never with the intention of restraining or punishing. The most susceptible area arises in our physical interactions. If we find ourselves grabbing someone, even with the best of intentions, then we are restraining. Our physical interactions need to be used solely to block violence, and the next moment we should be quickly considering how to prevent it. Verbal protection might involve playfully speaking with the person as we see signs of disorganization; "Hold on Matthew, don't forget what friendship means!" Then, this verbal interplay needs to be followed with a concrete demonstration such as transforming an intended blow into a handshake. Matthew is no fool. He feels that when two caregivers come near he is going to be pushed and pulled until he complies. Their hands and mouths symbolize forcefulness and overpowering. He rebels, while others simply obey like machines.

The caregiver who decided to try to be one with him watches his every movement to avoid representing domination, a "You do this, or else!" attitude. Her option was warm helping instead of demandingness, and when violence began to surge out of his anguish, she became calmer, more valuing, and ready to de-escalate it.

DOMINATIVE DIMENSION

There are other interactions that symbolize apartness and are expressed in domineering interactions. It is ironic that we often "treat" violence with violence, distance ourselves further from those who are already apart, and express coldness to those who need warmth. Death comes to the human spirit in many ways, often through subtle interactions that rust away at our being. Most often, these are done without our even knowing it, not only through punishment but through expressions that signal differentness, lessened value, and compliance as life's purpose rather than a deep desire to relate to others in a spirit of solidarity. These are as destructive as the more obvious practices that prevail, such as time out, taking away privileges, spankings, electric shock, seclusion, locking up people, and a host of other control mechanisms. All such interactions need to be eliminated if we want to teach feelings of companionship. The most common ones relate to the giving of demands and any interactions that are contingent and reflect a superior attitude.

Assisting Demandingly

Assisting demandingly refers to any caregiving interactions whose aim is to "help," but they are done in a cold, mechanistic, or authoritarian manner. They express a hierarchical, nonfraternal relationship toward the person. They indicate a degree of intolerance, impatience, and disregard. They give the feeling that control is the purpose rather than engagement. They are typically forceful in nature and over-focus on the mechanics of compliance instead of a flow of mutual participation. The caregiver feels compelled to make the person respond rather than empowering mutual participation. They symbolize a desire to impose correction and correctness rather than the use of participatory interactions as a means toward human valuing.

Physical demandingness refers to those acts of assistance using physical interventions that provoke or might provoke an emotional or physical tug-of-war, such as when the caregiver grabs a person's hand to force participation. The demanding nature of such assistance is seen in cries, screams, or any other form of rebellion that might result. Demandingness is expressed when the caregiver continues a resistance-provoking form of intervention rather than seeking a less demanding option. Our hands are like instruments that can be used to signal fear or kindness. This variable makes them symbols of force.

Verbal demandingness refers to the same as the above, except that the caregiver uses words or vocalizations such as "No, don't do that!" or "Pick it up!" in an authoritarian tone. These words or vocalizations give a feeling of inferiority. They could be easily substituted by less intrusive forms of communication, such as gestures or kind words. They include any cold verbal interactions.

Gestural demandingness refers to the same as the above, except that gesticulations replace words or physical contact, such as firmly pointing at an object, grimaces, or any other nonverbal expressions that lack warmth, focus on demand, or indicate an "I am the boss" attitude.

These interactions are probably the most common reason why we signal fear and even loathing in vulnerable people. They are generally very subtle things that we do, such as grabbing a person, taking someone's hand and forcing him or her to do something, giving demeaning or condescending instructions, and other interactions indicative of a feeling of apartness. Even when these are done in the name of helping the person, such interactions send clear messages that we are in authority and the focus is on obedience and compliance instead of companionship. They gnaw away at the human spirit and make the person feel that life is nothing more than rote compliance. Instead of a mutually valuing relationship, they value the caregiver instead of the person.

> Timothy's teacher just wants him to put the puzzle together. This seems simple enough to her, but she is thinking as much about him obeying her wish as completing the puzzle. When he refuses, she says, "Look at me! Do it now!" This makes the child more stubborn. He groans. She takes his hand forcefully and says, "I will help you." He feels her cold gaze and her forceful hand. They do the puzzle "together." She says, "Good job!" like a boss would say to a lowly employee. Neither smiles. Her words, gestures, and physical contact merge together to convey a strong message of oppression.

Demandingness takes many expressions, and it is critical to be sensitive to each form. Our words are commonly demanding, especially in their tone. "Pick it up!" can have various connotations depending on how we say it—how tolerant we are and if we are willing to become mutually engaged. It is impossible to show on paper what demandingness is. It can involve orders, but not all orders are demanding in the sense that they do not necessarily remove us from an equal relationship. "Why don't we pick up the paper?" is less demanding than the first request, and it can even become warm helping if accompanied by other words, gestures, or physical interactions that communicate, "I'll give you whatever help that you need; in fact, I'll go ahead and do it for you." Demandingness has much to do with our intentions. A good question to ask is, "Why am I interested in the other person doing this? To see that the individual obeys? Or to bring us closer together?"

Restraint, Reward, and Punishment

Restraint, reward and punishment refer to physical, verbal, or environmental actions that result in immobilization of the person by the caregiver or forced movement based on any form of compliance, treating the person as a being who has to earn reward or treating the person as a being who can be controlled or modified through reward or punishment. Their purposes are to control the person through a life based on contingency or control. These three types of interactions arise out of the belief that the powerful must modify the powerless. The caregiver operates under the belief that the human being is simply a mechanism that responds to the carrot and stick: "If you do good, you will be rewarded; if you do bad, you will be punished." Reward is viewed as the negation of the human condition when it is the basic procedure used to modify the other's behavior. Everything has to be earned and reward is delivered in a robot-like manner. Punishment is reward's twin. It is the bleaker side of the family of control. Restraint is often the last hope when the other two fail. It essentially says, "Since you do not respond to reward or punishment, we must lock you up, tie you up, or drug you." Restraint is seen in any use of any part of the caregiver's body or the surrounding environment that results in stopping a person's movement through grabbing or containing the person. It includes the use of any contingent orders designed to immobilize the person, such as orders to put one's hands down or in one's pockets, the use of time-out rooms, or the use of the environment to jail a person. It is also seen in the use of mechanical devices such as helmets and straitjackets.

Physical restraint refers to any bodily contact on the part of the caregiver that temporarily and, at least partially, incapacitates the person. It is beyond blocking in that it equates with physically stopping a person through holding onto a body part or putting one's weight on the body. It carries this act beyond the moment of potential harm and often escalates into violence. It becomes contingent and mechanistic in that it focuses solely on domination.

Verbal restraint refers to any verbal orders that have compliance as their purpose. It is seen in orders given in a planned or spontaneous way, such as "Hands down!" or verbal demands when a person is disruptive.

Environmental and mechanical restraint refers to any use of the setting designed to separate a person from the group, such as the use of separate rooms, screens, helmets, masks, or any other devices used to limit a person's movement. It is also characterized by the imposition of an object that can only be removed through the use of power, such as anchoring the person's chair to the floor.

Reward refers to patterns of caregiver interactions that predominantly center on a relationship based on control, even if they are positive and nonaversive. These interactions are seen in rigid procedures, wherein the person has to earn reward and the caregiver generally only gives positive attention for things earned. Like punishment, it views personkind as robot-like.

Punishment refers to caregiver interactions that focus on the use of any form of denial, withdrawal of privileges, or aversive therapy. These express a nonnurturing relationship and are cold and mechanistic. Punishment includes practices such as time out, overcorrection, verbal and physical reprimands, and the entire armamentarium of negative behavioral interventions.

Reward and punishment are characterized by any caregiver interactions that are based on the view that the person is nothing more than a machine, what some term as mere sets of stimuli and responses. It is dehumanizing to base our interactions on the notion that the center of the human condition is reward and punishment and that this rule is what brings about learning, including behavioral change. Doubtlessly, reward and punishment often work. But whether something works or not is not the issue. The central question is what kind of relationship do we want to create. Reward is different from valuing the person. It is scheduled and earned, applied to the person in a prescriptive format. It often involves the giving of material things, such as food or tokens.

It distances the caregiver from the person and emanates from an attitude that we are superior and that we have the power to modify the behavior of those who are alienated. Punishment is similar to reward. It is for deeds done, scheduled and applied as in a prescription. It involves verbal, physical, and gestural reprimands delivered in a broad number of ways. Most punishment is also accompanied at some point by various types of contingent reward. The idea is to use the "carrot" as much as possible, and, when that does not work, to use the "stick." Either view devalues the person. A life primarily comprised of reward or punishment is a life devoid of meaning.

> Daniel knows this when his caregivers take him into the seclusion room, or pounce on him on the floor, or give their mechanistic "Good job!" when he does something compliant. If he could talk, he would likely tell his caregivers to take their reward and punishment to hell. But he is unable to speak coherently, so his fists express his emptiness. And then hell visits him in the dreary seclusion room.
>
> He is supposed to be working in a "rehabilitation program" for homeless adults. He has no language and little desire to do what he is told. He might be mentally retarded, but nobody knows for sure. His shelter is similar to his workplace—sterile, devoid of laughter and friendship, and filled with caregiver voices and hands that seem to push and pull him. He keeps hearing the word *compliance*, spoken as if it were sacred. When he does some little chore he hears mechanistic voices say "Good job!" but when he refuses he inevitably hears, "Do it or we will have to make you!" Of course, he rebels. The tension escalates and a caregiver takes his arms and "guides" him through the steps. He becomes furious, fights, and swings his arms. Finally he is face down on the floor. His strong caregiver straddles his prone body and "helps" him complete the task. At the end he says "Good job!"

We have placed reward alongside punishment and restraint as an equally oppressive phenomenon because when interactions are delivered for the sake of a contingent consequence they are unilateral ways in which we communicate: "I am giving this to you because I have the power to modify your behaviors, and due to this I am over you." As a behavior modification practice, reward is an essential and ongoing pattern that puts the caregiver in a superior position. Even if it is given frequently, it encompasses a generally sterile or mechanistic relationship, and it dilutes unconditional interactions from which feelings of companionship arise.

CONCLUSION

We have a difficult and long road to journey. It requires ongoing questioning of what we are doing and why we are doing it. It asks us to change our direction by turning away from domination and embracing value-giving. It beckons us to reflect on our relationship with people who are engrossed in long patterns of rejection and being rejected. It asks us to be empathic with those who are vulnerable, sometimes for mysterious reasons, and with those who live anguished lives and are unable to reach out toward others until others reach out toward them. It asks us to participate in the feelings—the anguish and joy—of these persons who need caring and allow them to take part in our lives as well. It asks us to do away with straitjackets, helmets, and masks. It calls on us to abandon practices like placing people in time-out rooms and seclusion rooms. It requires us to opt out of an entire range of practices, from verbal reprimands to rewarding people only for deeds done.

Caregiving involves a commitment to give value in spite of rejection; it asks us to be tolerant, respectful, and persevering. It calls on us to teach others, even those who appear to be beyond the realm of human responsiveness, to both accept and reciprocate human valuing. It also asks us to bring about as much participation as we can, even in those who might seem totally unable or unwilling to become engaged. Most of all, it signifies change in us.

David refuses to participate; he bites, pulls out his hair, and throws furniture from one end of the room to the other. His caregiver says that he needs to be controlled. Thus, he is in a compliance-training program. He is given verbal instructions: "Tuck your shirt in . . . Make the bed . . . Hands down . . ." If he becomes more violent, he is brought to the floor and held "until calm." Each of these steps represents an almost countless number of domineering caregiver interactions, not just the gross instructions, but also the tone of voice, the grip of the hand, the coldness of the gaze, and the drive to overpower. If David is to change, his caregiver has to change.

The caregiver has to learn to dramatically increase his value-centered interactions. Over time, he begins to see David in a different light and values him as a friend. It is time to dry the dishes, but rather than saying, "David, go dry the dishes," he continues talking with David and holds out a dish towel. If David accepts it, fine. If not, the caregiver continues to dialogue while doing the dishes himself. He occasionally invites David to help. If David becomes angry, the caregiver continues to do the dishes. If necessary, he scoots the dishes away for a moment so they cannot be tossed. All along, valuing continues and the caregiver attempts to enable participation.

Even at the most violent moments, we need to concentrate our efforts on valuing instead of domination, keeping in check our primitive urge to overpower those who threaten us.

Anthony is in the midst of a fury, jumping up and down, throwing furniture, trying to bite and kick a caregiver. Two other staff members hear the screaming and enter the room ready to subdue him. Anthony sees them and becomes more violent. What is the option to treating violence with violence?

His caregiver tells the other two to back off since their presence symbolizes force and power. He decides to value Anthony as a father would his son. Nobody wants harm to come so he stands out of arm's reach; but he also wants Anthony to feel valued and nurtured. He speaks softly to him, "That's fine. I am not going to hurt you . . ." Anthony continues to escalate his violence. He slaps the caregiver once, then a second time. Yet the caregiver continues to encourage and protect. The rage slowly subsides. The caregiver has spent forty minutes protecting Anthony and himself while also trying to enable the slightest amount of participation from Anthony and continuing to speak softly to him. Since objects might be tossed, the caregiver uses his hands as the "activity," using them to reach out an ask for a handshake. This occurs during brief moments throughout the frenzy, but sufficient enough to let Anthony realize force will not follow violence.

This caregiver made a conscious decision to nurture Anthony instead of subduing him. The risk of harm was no greater, and perhaps less, in this nonviolent approach than in physically restraining Anthony. Reward would have been meaningless since Anthony was doing little to "earn" it. Punishment would have been a waste of energy since he was so emotionally disconnected at the moment. Restraint would have only told him to fight harder. So the caregiver's alternative was to value, warmly help, and elicit valuing from Anthony. Whether Daniel, David, or Anthony, our role is to cease dominating individuals and practice valuing them instead.

Chapter 4
THE PERSON'S INTERACTIONS
Union versus Apartness

We have looked at ourselves and examined the many interactions we need to consider in order to become more value-centered and less domineering. Turning our attention to marginalized persons, we can see similar interactional patterns. Their aggression, self-harm, or withdrawal represent apartness—a surrender to anguish, meaninglessness, and choicelessness. Our dominative interactions compound them. Our central role is not to find ways to get rid of their behavior problems, but to enable the learning of accepting and returning unconditional valuing and engagement. As we do this, feelings of apartness disappear. Behavioral difficulties do not exist as much as interactional ones, and we play a central role in the presence or absence of violence in others through our everyday interactions. There is no form of aggression, self-injury, or withdrawal that is not related to and influenced by our interactions. If the person is slapping or hitting, we have to ask what we are doing. Are our words demanding? Is our gaze devaluing? Is our tone authoritarian or cold? The homeless person on the street falls deeper into despair with our frozen stares. The woman with schizophrenia who is grabbed by a caregiver loses more of life's meaning. The child spanked by a parent senses more loneliness. And although some persons are born in disharmony, our commitment needs to be centered on teaching even those most distant persons to be part of family and community life. The process, then, needs to start with us and move both ourselves and others toward companionship. Our purpose is to diminish a sense of being apart from others by establishing feelings of union with us and others.

VULNERABILITY

Persons with behavioral difficulties are vulnerable. Some have more difficulty reflecting on their actions, understanding them, and acquiring a range of social-emotional skills to deal with them. This is sometimes due to inborn disabilities, such as mental retardation or some forms of mental illness. Others risk developing feelings of apartness due to social-political circumstances, such as those that arise from poverty. Whether caused internally or externally, our responsibility is to help each person enter into a change process with us. In fact the weakest among us need the most emotional support. Regardless of the cause, vulnerability is exacerbated by the world's lack of response to basic human needs and its shunting aside those who are disobedient, rebellious, nonproductive, or just different. The perception of differentness often equates with worthlessness and leads to segregation and conditions based on control instead of companionship. The end result is violence to self or others, for example, the violence of punching someone, slamming one's head on the floor, or simply withdrawing from human contact. Marginalization is a life condition in which we push vulnerable people to the outer limits of society. It gives rise to a feeling of isolation and meaninglessness, with no connections with others. An emerging sense of union beckons longingly for valuing and being valued, a condition in which the other feels safe, wants to be with others, and receives and reciprocates valuing.

The presence of behavioral difficulties does not mean that caregivers have not shown much love, affection, and warmth. Indeed, often a child or adult has very problematic behaviors in spite of these traits. Countless numbers of parents show profound love and yet see their child develop severe behavioral problems. A

basic factor that is forgotten is that bonded relationships are mutual and reciprocal. Love given does not necessarily mean love
returned. A parent can pour love and affection on a child and still
see that child withdraw or become violent. For many vulnerable
people, such as those with autism, we have to literally teach the
reciprocation of valuing. The key is both love given and love
elicited. The central question is often not what the caregiver has or
has not done or what amount of warmth and affection has been
given; rather, it revolves around the person's vulnerabilities and
our focus. We can show deep affection and care and still not seek
its reciprocation. We can overprotect because we do not know
what else to do, or we can miss seeing the person's difficulty all
together until it has mushroomed, sometimes seemingly beyond
hope. In addition, many caregivers become so enthralled with
teaching the acquisition of skills that they forget about or diminish
the importance of emotions, or they become enchanted with the
notion of compliance and abandon nurturing. Our challenge is to
teach the person to come to us by us going to them. We need to
melt the ice that has frozen over their hearts. Once thawed, they
will begin to fulfill the longing for union. This is a most difficult
process. Most of the work, discipline, and patience falls on our
shoulders.

A psychology of interdependence is based on the belief that all
humans long for meaning, companionship, choice, and freedom.
For those who are marginalized, this search is more laborious
since they have been pushed to the very edges of family and
community life. Their hearts try to grasp meaning, but it eludes
them. Their minds seek ways out of anguish, but poverty and
segregation has fallen over them like a shroud. And choice becomes a hollow sound in a world of behavior modification. Some
say that skill acquisition and compliance are the most fundamen-
tally necessary elements in family and community life; indeed, it is
important that each person develop his or her talents to the maximum and that individuals learn to respect others and live within
prosocial norms. But these elements are not the cornerstones of
the human condition. They are secondary and can evolve as

beneficial side effects of feeling in harmony with others. Certainly, they can be achieved through control. But they can also emerge out of the mutual respect and self-worth that is inherent in a spirit of companionship. As this takes root, mutual respect, sharing, and other socializing interactions spring forth. Our option is to generate and nurture this process and watch these critical elements of the human spirit blossom.

The longing for feelings of companionship resides within all people; yet in some its emergence is frozen, and no matter how hard the person tries, the thickened ice cannot thaw without warm help. Feelings of division arise out of domination, and this thickens iced-over hearts even more. Valuing is the intense sunshine that showers warmth and melts the wintery feelings of apartness. Union with others can be seen when individuals gradually begin to accept valuing, return it, become engaged, and share with others. It involves a physical proximity as well as an emotional coming together. It is eloquent in its simplicity, with smiles, nods of friendship, joshing, laughing, communicating sorrows and joys, and helping others. We have already touched on the importance of helping the person learn to return valuing and that this reciprocation equalizes and transforms the relationship. This soon evolves into natural expressions. We no longer have to elicit it; it flows out spontaneously. Sharing is another critical factor, not only interacting with a particular caregiver, but learning to reach out to others. This feeling of mutuality occurs within the context of engagement with others and an expanding sense that being together is good in and of itself.

RESIGNIFYING REALITY

The world takes on distinct meanings depending on each person's reality, vulnerabilities, talents, history, and support networks. These meanings are filled with signs and symbols. To resignify is to give new meanings. We need to initiate a process in which the meaning of companionship takes root and apartness disappears. A homeless person might see most others as oppressors; an abused child might cringe when just seeing an adult approach; a retarded adult, upon seeing others working and playing, might feel saddened by the feeling that such fulfillment is beyond reach. These old meanings need to be discarded. We have the responsibility to introduce new feelings through our interactions so that the marginalized person begins to feel one with us, united instead of apart, embracing instead of avoiding, engaged instead of obedient, and valued instead of controlled.

Our reality and that of the other person need to be given new meanings. Different signs and symbols need to fill an absurd world. These meanings are embedded within and between people and translate into how we perceive ourselves and others, how the other sees us, and how their interpretations transform themselves into actions. When we feel no companionship toward the aggressive person, our interactions are not able to convey warmth and authenticity. Our words reflect apartness and our hands are seen as aggressive. Likewise, the marginalized person has deeply rooted meanings. These weigh on the person like stones. The person views his or her self as worthless and looks upon us as agents of force and control. When the person sees us, it is better to avoid him or her rather than reach out or to simply obey rather than dialogue.

In order to bring new meanings to the human condition, we

Resignifying Reality	
From	*To*
Apartness ⟶	Union
Avoidance ⟶	Reaching out
Compliance ⟶	Engagement
Control ⟶	Unconditional valuing

need to assume the responsibility for our own change as well as an initial commitment to enable feelings of union in the other. This interpretation of behavioral difficulties leads us to see the other in the shadow of anguish. Even if aggression, self-injury, or withdrawal appear to be volitional, we need to understand each person's history and translate this into the here and now. The new meanings that we elicit are indicative of companionship, a relationship based on mutuality, marked by warmth and openness and centered on unconditional valuing. The challenge is not to modify observable behaviors alone, but to transform the very essence of the human condition and to change the reality of marginalization.

Union

We have seen the principle value-centered interactions to which we need to be committed. Now let us examine the other side of the interactional nature of caregiving. These factors help the person learn to express companionship and create new meanings in life based on feelings of interdependence. They represent our helping others center their life valuing. And this is what brings about union. They necessitate active caregiver involvement and do not simply evolve; rather, we have to teach them. To establish feelings of union, we need to concentrate our efforts on teaching the person to reciprocate our valuing, to initiate it on their own, to become engaged with us, and to share these feelings with others.

Union	
• Value reciprocation	• Value-initiation
• Engagement	• Sharing

Value Reciprocation

Value reciprocation refers to any interactions on the part of
the person that express or are indicative of the person's return of
valuing toward the caregiver who is eliciting it. These are related
to the caregiver's seeking smiles, handshakes, hugs, and any facial,
corporal, or verbal interactions related to returning signs of union. These help to equalize and democratize the relationship so
that the other is not a perpetual recipient, but an active participant
in a value-centered life condition. Our task is not only to give
valuing, but to teach its return.

> *Physical reciprocation* refers to the person giving any
> physical contact representative of valuing the caregiver, such
> as handshakes, hugs, patting one's hand or arm, and any
> similar contacts. It includes even slight, almost impercept-
> ible, interactions such as a brief touch of a finger in an
> attempt to respond to a handshake.
> *Verbal reciprocation* refers to the same as the above, ex-
> cept that words or vocalizations are used. These include
> words of praise given by the person or sounds that indicate
> pleasure, happiness, and joy related to the caregiver's pres-
> ence or participation with the caregiver. They also include
> dialogue, expressing feelings, and the sharing of hopes and
> anguish.
> *Gestural reciprocation* refers to the same as the above,
> except gestures replace words or touch. These are seen in
> actions such as smiles, gazing warmly, and any other bodily
> movements indicating a sense of being valued or safe.

Giving value to the other person also assumes a commitment
to elicit it. As we do this, we are teaching the person to return our
valuing. This results in the emergence of a mutual relationship in
which the other begins to express signs of bonding. It conveys the
feeling that the person is entering into a spirit of dialogue. In the

beginning, reciprocation is often minute movements away from previous patterns.

> When the caregiver places his hand in Anthony's, he is elicit-
> ing valuing from him, and the gradual willingness to allow this is
> the start of reciprocation. The smile that arises when he touches
> Anthony's face is an integral part of learning to reach out. In spite
> of Anthony's fury, the caregiver gives unconditional valuing and
> expresses nurturing. At every change the caregiver seeks any slight
> reciprocation. He touches Anthony's hand and face, asks for a
> handshake and a smile, and talks to him about being friends. Anth-
> ony begins to feel safe, accepts the touch, and finally gives a hand-
> shake. He glances quizzically and shows the faintest smile.

Value-Initiating

Value-initiating refers to the same phenomena as the above, except these interactions are initiated spontaneously. They can appear apart from value reciprocation or within it. They often start to occur once the person begins to sense the meaning of the elicited reciprocation and indicate an internalization of the good-ness of being with the caregiver. When we ask for a handshake and the person also responds with a warm gaze, the latter would be interpreted as the initiation of a form of value-giving. This is no small matter; it signals the start of a different relationship—one based on emerging companionship.

The initiation of valuing toward the caregiver indicates that the person is moving beyond mere reciprocation and starting to naturally express warmth, affection, and authentic friendship. These interactions arise on their own and do not require the caregiver's seeking them. They mean that feelings of safety and security are emerging, engagement with the caregiver is becoming an important and significant dimension in the person's life, and being valued and giving value is starting to take root at the center of the human condition. They are the clearest sign and symbol of the formation and equalization of the relationship and signal the advent of interdependence. We have to take care to be sensitive to these expressions and be aware of their importance so that we might continue to enable and encourage them.

> As Anthony begins to reciprocate hints of smiles and hand-shakes, the probability increases that these phenomena will become a natural part of his interaction with those who accept and value him. The hours and days wear on and he becomes more ready and willing to reciprocate valuing. The caregiver asks for a handshake and Anthony offers his hand, smiles, and embraces the caregiver. Reciprocation is starting to become natural and, indeed, Anthony goes beyond that which is sought. One act multiplies into another and another. The unexpected smiles and embraces tell the caregiver that Anthony is, indeed, becoming a companion.

Engagement

Engagement refers to the person's willingness and desire to be with and participate with the caregiver. It is conveyed in interactions such as moving closer, paying attention longer, working together, playing together, listening intently, and using one's talents. It relates secondarily to the acquisition of skills and fulfilling responsibilities. These begin to emerge as the person feels secure and accepts our unconditional valuing. Engagement enables the person to express feelings of being with the other. It is like a bridge that links us with marginalized others. This bridging is often done in the face of rebellion or near total withdrawal. So we need to effectuate it by putting aside any focus on compliance. The fact that a person might know how to do something is irrelevant. The desire to participate with us is the key element. If we react with observations such as, "He knows how to do this so he should!" then we leave the person floundering in the backwaters of isolation. Our task is to enable engagement regardless of the person's abilities or skills. If the person refuses to cook supper, the question here is not culinary skills, but the emergence of the feeling of being with us. We need to give whatever help might be necessary to bring about participation, so we can nurture this feeling.

Doing tasks together is a vehicle for this. In essence, as we seek to bring about participation, day-to-day activities serve as the structure within which engagement occurs, such as when the mother invites the child to wash dishes with her, when the father helps his child clean his bedroom, when the teacher sits with the student, or when the group home worker goes shopping with the resident. Each of these activities has the potential of bringing the other closer to us. However, if this does not happen, we need to enable it slowly by giving whatever amount of help might be necessary. Engagement is broken into two subvariables, with the caregivers helping the person or without any direct help. We encourage maximum personal development, yet, especially at the start, it is critical that we lend as much help as necessary, even if we do nearly everything.

With help refers to any level of physical, verbal, or gest-ural assistance that the caregiver lends to the person in order to bring about participation. Regardless of the person's abil-ities, the caregiver does this by doing activities with or even for the person as long as the individual is at least a passive participant.

Without help refers to participation with the caregiver or on one's own with no special supports necessary. This is seen when the person is able to continue participating when the caregiver is not present or does not have to offer any unique help.

By enabling and facilitating participation, we help the person start to perceive being with others as a central part of the human condition. A feeling of solidarity emerges. The person begins to participate in activities and tasks throughout the flow of the day, not due to any feeling of compliance, but due to the evolution of a spirit of being together with the one enabling it. Its strongest indicator is when we are with the person, doing a task together, and dialoguing. This signifies that companionship is solidifying.

Most hospitals, institutions, work training centers, shelters, and special schools focus on rehabilitation through learning an occupation or acquiring skills. Indeed, it is good to work and develop and express our talents. But for most marginalized people, work or schooling is, at best, secondary. Low pay, no benefits, and long hours of heavy work do little to lift up the human spirit. More importantly, a life without significant others shatters the person's ability to develop individual talents. Sitting in a classroom and becoming literate are important, but need to be considered within the context of the person's emotional needs. Houses, cottages, and special residential units devoid of friendship do little to spark the human spirit. These are made of bricks and mortar; a home is made of love and companionship. It does little good to teach someone to wash clothing or prepare meals if that person cannot reach out and honor those around.

Our option for a culture of life leads us to seek engagement with the person instead of using skill acquisition or obedience as a central element in the development of value-centered relationships. In many settings, individuals are trained to comply, but not to know one another; to obey, but not to respect and trust. Engagement starts with us using ourselves as the reason for coming together. Because individuals often initially rebel against engagement, we need to enable it through our participation with the person and ongoing valuing.

What about someone with severe disabilities who can hardly move or understand his surroundings? Is it possible to establish a feeling of engagement and bring about participation in those with the profoundest mental retardation?

> Kathleen was born with profound mental retardation and died when she was two years old. She was unable to suck, chew, or swallow. She was blind and deaf, and she was never able to sit up by herself. Although she spent her time arched in a frequent state of seizure activity, her mother and father assumed that she could learn to participate in life in her own unique way. They embraced her as a full human being and taught their two other children that Kathleen was equal to everyone. They understood that their baby's worth would have to be seen in another dimension; she was still a complete, loving human being. Her parents taught her to move

her tiny hand when it was in theirs and to smile and move her tongue as if kissing. This was her embrace and her demonstration of affection—not much, but more than many humans are willing to express. Her struggle to do this much was her labored way of being engaged. This mutuality ended with her death. But while living, she was able to show oneness with her parents and siblings. How did her parents teach this?

They spent hours with the baby, placing their fingers in her hand, valuing her, caressing her, and encouraging the slightest movement. They kissed her on her cheek and encouraged the tiniest expressions of warmth and love. They touched her lips and helped her move them over their fingers as her kiss. Her sounds also began to "speak" messages of the desire for and affirmation of union. This infant required much, but also gave much. Her mother said, "She is both a burden and a joy. A burden because of the constant care; a joy because the slightest sign of her affection, her acknowledgement of our presence, and her movement toward us was a moment of celebration."

The desire to be with us and reaching out toward us indicate that the person feels safe and secure. The act of participating with us is a sign of companionship. It is a moving toward the other in a spirit of solidarity. Human engagement means that the other is entering into our life space because there is an emerging sense of oneness. Without it, valuing occurs in a vacuum and is one-sided. We need to be at the person's side, not because we are important, but because we are equal. Learning to be with us is learning to become engaged, both for the other and ourselves. Doubtlessly, we have to enable the evolution of individual talents, but within the context of learning human engagement. This indicates the elaboration of feelings of connection with us as sources of valuing and its reciprocation.

Sharing

We need to expand this initial relationship to others by bringing our newly-formed relationship to a broader number of other individuals. Sharing generates this process. Instead of downward relationships, as seen in a staff-to-client world, the purpose of sharing is to create a circle of friends that expands outward. Old-fashioned sewing circles are examples of what this process looks like. People come together to make a beautiful quilt, but all the while the group is dialoguing. Another example is barn raising, when farmers come together to help a neighbor in distress by using construction to express unity. In urban settings, volunteers join hands to rehabilitate deserted buildings for human habitation. Also, a teacher may ask her students to show and tell about their prized possessions. The busy hands, the productivity, and the telling are reasons to come together. Sharing breaks up the tendency to live independent, but parallel, lives. It is the soup kitchen where the homeless work together, the group home where all are learning to live together, and the classroom where the children are helped to reach out to one another.

Emotional strength and stability increase as the circle of companions broadens. A key factor is to teach the other to share and reach out, first to us, then to others. Sharing involves any interactions on the part of the person that indicate participation with or expressing value toward persons other than the primary caregiver. These can be self-initiated or self-elicited. We have the responsibility to encourage the person to seek friendship with others since friendship does not automatically transfer to others; it needs to be extended. Additionally, we need to make sure that the person doesn't become overdependent on us since this stagnates maximum fulfillment.

Sharing can occur in two ways: through doing tasks together or through valuing others. In the first, we use common activities as vehicles to bring others around us and the person whom we are helping. This concrete approach is a good way to start the sharing process. The second way is more complex and involves teaching the group to value one another. These two processes are often combined, the first giving a structure, the second deepening the meaning.

Task-centered sharing is the process of using activities to bring persons together who are outside the primary dyad. It is seen, for example, when a caregiver encourages two or three individuals help each other prepare a meal together.

Person-centered sharing is the same process, but with a focus on teaching the participants to give honor and respect to one another. It is seen, for example, when the caregiver helps a person shake someone else's hand: "John, why don't you shake Anthony's hand and thank him for helping us!" or when the caregiver facilitates a dialogue among the participants.

Anthony learned to become engaged with the caregiver and then share with others. As he began to feel safe with them, the caregiver focused more on teaching him to reach out to the others, talk with them, and thank them for their help.

Little Kathleen learned to share and extend her feelings beyond those she felt toward her parents by reaching out to her brother and sister. Her mother would often have them help in feeding, bathing, and dressing. More importantly during these times, Kathleen made sure that their interactions were similar to hers, valuing her with caresses, hugs, and kisses; encouraging the baby to make slight movements to show her love; and, teaching other family members these nuances. As simple as these movements were, they were Kathleen's way of showing love and sharing her fulfillment.

Distancing interactions increase over time unless we reach out and teach others to become engaged with and participate with us. These interactions begin to disappear in direct relation to the formation of companionship, first with a significant other, then with others. Aggression, self-injury, and withdrawal are the opposite of value-giving and its reciprocation. They are contradictions of human engagement and sharing. As we teach value-centered interactions, the person begins to learn to reject violence, disruptiveness, and destruction in his or her relationships with those who are just. We need to be keenly aware of the importance of extending these feelings beyond the person's relationship with us in order that he or she construct the strongest social network possible. The ability to reach out toward others strengthens emotional fortitude and the ability to face life's vicissitudes. The first steps toward sharing are difficult. The person often passes through the same fear, distancing, and meaninglessness with others as with the first caregiver. Then, when the person develops a feeling of companionship with the caregiver, the person feels there is little reason to inch beyond this one relationship. So we need to invite others to participate and facilitate the expansion of these feelings.

Apartness

A culture of death* gives birth to isolation, loneliness, and marginalization. These are expressed in violence–the hatred and fear conveyed through aggression, the suicidal attempts of self-injury, and the despair of withdrawal. Apartness is what behaviorists would term a tendency toward maladaptive behavior, but it is much deeper than what we observe. It resides in the inner heart and eats away at the anguished spirit. Getting rid of observable behaviors does not solve the mysteries of the heart; it only serves to mask them, often in a frozen state of obedience. Apartness comes from moment to moment, ordinary, gnawing-away feelings such as those seen when caregivers focus on obedience. "Hands down! Sit!" might seem like a good thing for a caregiver to demand of a marginalized person, but for the latter, such commands instill fears that multiply and accumulate until their weight crushes any desire to be with others. Our dominative interactions ac-

---

*A culture of death is based on a spirit of individualism and independence instead of solidarity and interdependence. It devalues anyone who is unable to fend for himself or herself. It is seen in the ways in which the poor, the mentally ill, the aged, and the mentally retarded are treated. Unable to produce, they are separated from community life, and they are expected to obey their caregivers. If the marginalized are disruptive, their behaviors are modified so that they comply with social norms. A culture of death is expressed in cold and sterile caregiver interactions that empty the marginalized of any feelings of solidarity.

Apartness	
•Aggression	•Self-injury
•Active withdrawal	•Passive withdrawal

cumulate in a pattern that tells the person there is no hope for union and that aggression or self-injury is the best way to deal with increasing isolation.

Distancing behaviors are any actions or interactions that might potentially result in physical or emotional harm to self or others. They indicate emotional homelessness in that they serve to remove the person from engagement and participation, whether through withdrawal, self-injury, or aggression. They connote fear of others and loudly proclaim the lack of adequate valuing and its perceived meaninglessness. These behaviors are signs and symbols of the lack of union and the presence of feelings of oppression. Our task is to take away their meaning through our value-centered interactions. Our designification of these gives more power to our valuing. Again, we can get rid of such behaviors through force or control. But our option is to create new interactional patterns. These then are replaced by valuing, its reciprocation, and engagement.

Aggression refers to acts of violence or attempts at these acts. They include cursing, hitting, biting, kicking, scratching, pulling hair, spitting at others, vomiting on them, throwing objects at them, pinching, ripping clothing, poking others, and any other forms of verbal or physical violation.

Self-injury refers to phenomena such as the above except that they are directed at the self. These include pinching self, hitting any part of the body with any other part of the body, cutting self, pulling one's own hair, scratching self, banging one's head, tearing one's skin, inserting objects into the body, eating dangerous objects, slapping self, becoming dependent on chemicals, and any other form of self-harm, including attempts at suicide.

Active withdrawal refers to the person's actions or inter-actions that result in physical or emotional movement away from participation and result in disruption. These include running from the caregiver, sliding onto the floor, climbing upon chairs or ledges, stomping feet, pounding hands on tables, seeking out food or liquids instead of participating, and any other forms of physically removing self from en-gagement with the caregiver.

Passive withdrawal refers to the person's actions that re-sult in nonparticipation, without necessarily disrupting or harming others. These include sleeping; feigning sleep; crossing one's arms; looking away; body-rocking; licking spittle; waving hands, arms, or objects; hair twirling; hand- or arm-flapping; talking to self; mouthing objects or fingers; covering one's face or body; rituals with fingers, hands, or mouth; rumination; or regurgitation.

These behaviors are emotional ways of distancing self from others or drawing caregivers to self in the faint hope of attention. They are sometimes indicative of self-survival, even in the midst of the paradox of harm itself. Indeed, for many, punishment can be their reward since even negative contact can be seen as better than nothing. They are sometimes suicidal, giving up hope, sending a signal that "I am nobody" in a world devoid of meaning, friend-ship, and fulfillment. They involve complex ways of dealing with a reality they perceive as being void of affectionate contact with others. Through these behaviors, the person feels no value in being with others, and, when approached, refuses to accept val-uing or become engaged. Or they serve as ways to draw others toward self in a call for help.

Commonly we use phrases such as "inability to attend," "fail-ure to comply," and "incorrect participation" to throw the blame on the marginalized person. Yet before ridiculing the other we need to look at our own beliefs and practices. Aggression includes all those interactions that are symbolic of the person's moving away from us: swearing, demanding, hitting, biting, kicking, scratching, throwing, destroying property, and on down the list. They represent the person's total rejection of us and reflect the fear and absurdity inherent in the person's world. The twin of aggression is self-injury. Some persons turn inward and violate their own being. It is more tragic than aggression since it is an attack upon the self and is the essence of human anguish and feelings of meaninglessness. While some attack others or harm themselves, still others learn to simply withdraw from human contact, sometimes quite actively and at other times passively. Passive withdrawal is just as devastating to the human spirit. However, because it is often not so disruptive to others, it is frequently overlooked as a serious interactional difficulty. In reality, it is as indicative of apartness as any form of aggression or self-injury.

Anthony and Kathleen had their unique ways of expressing apartness. Anthony discovered violence toward others as his way of confronting years of caregiver coldness and demands. His fists struck with force. And even though often forced to comply, he was never engaged. He had no regard for his caregivers and knew aggression was a strong option. Little Kathleen was different. She simply could not reach out, so she tended to withdraw. Her mother had to dig deeply to find the seedlings of oneness with her. Her passive withdrawal left her helpless. Each person finds a unique way to deal with a world perceived as absurd or one in which reaching out is impossible without help. Our challenge is to bring meaning and warm help to these realities.

CONCLUSION

We are called on to fulfill a twofold responsibility: to decrease our domination and increase our valuing. Through this we help others move away from feelings of apartness and toward those of union. This mutual change process is complex and our responsibility is great. We are enablers and facilitators in the marginalized person's movement toward companionship. Our central concern should not revolve around the behavior problem, but on the reciprocation of our valuing, engagement with us, and sharing with others. A psychology of interdependence encompasses interactional change, a process in which our interactions are interwoven within the marginalized person's. Obviously, control and contingency procedures can bring about change in observable behaviors. But our purpose is the elaboration of feelings of companionship and the creation of mutual change in what is seen and felt within and between ourselves and marginalized people.

Chapter 5
DIALOGUE
The Expression of Human Valuing

We have looked into the purposes of caregiving and the factors that comprise a relationship based on companionship. We have emphasized the need to establish this as our fundamental goal and have spelled out three initial processes that need to be taught if this purpose is to unfold: the establishment of feelings of safety and security, engagement, and valuing. We have also described the main factors that make up the beginning of this relationship, both in ourselves and in the other, and have emphasized the mutual change that transpires. Questioning our relationship and putting valuing at the center of our day-to-day interactions essentially leads us to a newer and deeper practice that we call dialogue. Since human relationships and interactions are so intertwined with mutual feelings, dialogue with the marginalized person facilitates and centers the entire process. It is the core that permeates a value-centered relationship.

DIALOGUE

Dialogue is the energizing force of caregiving, especially among those who are disconnected from others and distance themselves through acts of aggression, self-injury, and withdrawal. It resignifies the relationship by placing ongoing valuing and sharing at the center of all interactions. It brings our life into the other's, therefore it is the ultimate expression of union. Because the distanced person needs an ongoing source of unconditional valuing, dialogue is critical since it provides a constant source of warmth, affection, and positive regard.

Dialogue has a multitude of expressions. It starts with the communication of feelings through physical, verbal, and gestural expressions. When we speak, we are opening up ourselves—communicating our happiness, our understanding of sorrow, our interests, and our reality. Dialogue involves a weaving in of words about the other's reality and the commonality in the yet-to-be-established relationship. Its intensity is modulated and sensitive to the emotional state of the other. When the other is nervous, we speak serenely. When the other is angry, we speak nurturing words. When the other is withdrawn, our words are exceptionally warm. Dialogue includes stories that teach the other new life meanings, including abstract stories, such as the feelings inherent in friendship and being at home. It helps the person imagine and articulate what a just and equal relationship and life condition might consist of. It expresses sentiments related to safety and security, the goodness of doing things together, and the centrality of valuing and being valued. Dialogue is never contingent; it is always given. It never ceases; it continues during good moments

---

Dialogue is
- Words shared about ourselves
- Words shared about the other
- At times animated, at times serene
- Silent expressions of friendship
- Story-telling
- Life directing
- Observations of the human condition
- Encouragement to feel safe, to participate, and to value self and others
- Unconditional and ongoing
- Linked with mutual participation, and engagement

and bad. It can be silent, but it always exudes warmth and mutuality, whether with words or other human expressions.

Most often, we have been trained to deliver reward rather than enter into the marginalized person's world, let alone allowing someone into ours. The contingent delivery of reward such as "Good job!" is a mechanistic way of interacting that brings little feeling of humanity. It might modify behaviors, due to the lack of any other positive interactions, but it is devoid of warmth and authenticity. It leaves the person as a perpetual recipient and discouraged from actively giving self to others. It tells the person that life is based on what is seen, not what is felt.

Caregivers who dedicate themselves to working among the most severely mentally retarded, mentally ill, and other oppressed individuals know how difficult dialogue can be. Due to the severity of the marginalization, we often start with only unilateral communication. There is generally little or no meaningful response. Indeed, rejection is often the rule. We have to be willing and ready to deal with this frustration. Dialogue is the transmission of empathy and understanding, the sharing of our experiences, and the revelation of joys and sorrow. This spirit helps move us away from the attitude that we are better or that the person should heed our kindness. We need to show a profound sense of brotherhood and sisterhood. Ironically, it often has to be initiated in the face of nonresponsiveness; but this is an element of our own change process that firms up our tolerance, patience, and giving without initially receiving.

Creating Dialogue

It is quite challenging to create a spirit of dialogue with anyone; it is harder still with someone pushed to the edge of life. With little or no meaningful reaction, it might even seem contradictory. However, if mutuality is to emerge, it is our responsibility to lay the foundation for this spirit regardless of reactions, appearances, diagnoses, or treatment mandates. Even though it may appear totally devoid of receptivity at the beginning, we assume that all people have an inherent hunger for feelings of warmth and engagement. Dialogue involves the mobilization of feelings of authenticity and honesty. Since the person has no reason to feel any of these, we need to care enough to generate them. This can only come about if we ourselves feel a longing for companionship and commence to transmit it, even though we might feel that it is meaninglessness. Dialogue's beginning is akin to planting seeds in a hostile earth: The rocks and weeds have to be cleared, and the soil has to be tilled. Only then can the seeds take root.

Unfortunately, we are accustomed to using mechanistic and frigid language, often in the form of demands and step-by-step prescribed communication. This translates into a monologue with the person that is heard time and again: "Pick it up . . . Hands down . . . Look at me . . . Good job . . . Good hands down . . . Good looking at me . . ." Such commentaries serve to further separate the person from meaningful relationships because they proliferate apartness. Dialogue has nothing to do with the expression of commands or verbal reward. It has to do with feelings of union rather than obedience, mutuality rather than mockery, and the elicitation and celebration of warm affection rather than the deepening of feelings of loneliness and isolation.

Dialogue is much more than a feeling of rapport with the person. It necessitates our total awakening from the start and the gradual awakening of the other person; our understanding what segregation, restraint, and punishment lead a person to become; sharing this with the person; and helping the person define reality. It is an awakening of our consciousness regarding our values toward ourselves, and it asks us to help the other imagine what the human condition could be. This raising of consciousness is useless if it is not accompanied by our commitment to act on it.

> Ted stands screaming and lashing out. He yells, "Want to go home! Want to go home!" The words echo throughout the workplace. He tears his shirt off. The caregiver continues her dialogue. He tips over tables and chairs and threatens the caregiver with his

swinging arms. Since she knows Ted and feels sisterly toward him, she realizes that the absence of feeling at "home" is the theme that destroys his being. She talks with him about the meaning of home, even though he continues to thrash about and scream. She speaks softly of homelessness and friendship and of her own longing for being at home. She speaks of his pain at not feeling at home. She protects herself from his flailing arms and thrashing feet. She remains nurturing while resuming an activity that he had tossed on the floor. Every now and then she helps him participate. He begins to calm. She continues sharing and doing the task for him, then with him. He sits, rocks, and moves his hands toward her as she reaches out toward him. This simple physical extension is a sign of the beginning of his dialogue. No words, just warm movement.

The feeling of oneness goes far beyond a caregiver–client relationship. It has to do with the responsibility of entering into the person's world, feeling the anguish and absurdity, sensing the fears and rejection, empathizing with these, and looking for a common ground for sharing. It has to do with the installation of hope regarding the meaningfulness of life and the spirit of companionship that rests within us. Ted's caregiver senses this and, in spite of his anger, emboldens herself to stay with him and engage him. Throughout these difficult moments, she expresses unconditional valuing in her words and actions.

When Ted screams, "Go home, go home, go home!" we need to sense his urge to be with those who are warm, the reflection of our own presence as meaningless or frightening, and our own longing to feel at home. Indeed, those words and acts, screams and

---

The process of creating dialogue involves
- Creating a feeling of oneness within ourselves
- Gaining insight into the person's history and social reality
- Interacting with the person in an open and honest way
- Interpreting what the person's interactions are saying
- Searching for those themes that are congruent with our own reality so that we might better communicate mutual feelings

shoves, and moans and hits that are often called behavioral problems are Ted's only instruments for expression in an otherwise
disharmonious world. We need to understand the confusion and
absurdity that swirls around and encircles him as well as the potential for solidarity. Dialogue serves to solidify the relationship—
slowly, with difficulty, but inevitably.

The creation of a feeling of oneness emerges from our values.
This means that we see Ted as one with us in spite of his behavior.
This leads us to accept him as our brother. The more we know
about his reality, the more we will be able to dialogue. Our interactions should be frank and free, clearly avoiding denigrations,
commands, and any focus on obedience and control. We need to
be sharp observers of the human condition because in the beginning the person will find little or no meaning in the dialogue. We
have to read the nonverbal communication as much as listen to the
verbal. This metacommunication—the combined expression of
the person's emotional, cognitive, and physical communication—
speaks an eloquent and complex language. We need to be open to
the person's tone, look, and movements as well as words and
sounds. This interpretation forms the theme for the dialogue. The
individual will eventually give subtle expressions of oneness: slight
smiles and gazes, changes in tone, increased engagement, and
more comfortable physical movements. Finally, we have to understand and share our own personal and social reality because dialogue is mutual. Unless we know and give of ourselves, it can easily
revert to one-sided, irrelevant, or condescending commentaries.

Initial distancing interactions, such as Ted's, are symbolic of
parallel lives—ours and his. We have to bring or life together with
his. To be parallel is to exist apart. It is a sign of solitude. We and
the other can easily fall into a pattern of separate existence: caregivers over clients, individual plans that do not reflect the whole
person, separate meals, separate breaks, the posting of rules, contingent reward, and other acts that we use to differentiate ourselves. It is impossible to create a shared life condition when we
regard ourselves as better. When the marginalized person looks at
us, we need to recognize that our human presence does not signify

any mutuality and find ways to shatter these difference. We can easily pass through the same feelings upon beholding the person. Indeed, we can be filled with fear, afraid of being hurt, rejected, or humiliated. Part of our responsibility is to transcend these feelings and remain harmonious and congruent with our beliefs by transforn.ing these into a feeling of union in spite of the near total emotional segregation and by breaking away from any feelings of superiority in favor of equality.

Themes

Our dialogue's themes need to be congruent with our own lives and the person's. For example, the person who is screaming that he or she does not want to participate might be trying to communicate that being with us signals fear of our force. We might talk about what being together means, that we are just as afraid as the person is, or that together we can protect one another. These themes require us to use our imagination and transcend the ordinary and the expected. They are often life-directing and involve helping the person learn rules for living. As the caregiver extends her hand to Ted, she might say, "Now, Ted! This means we are friends!" This helps define the establishment of feelings of companionship within an initial context of despair, hatred, and confusion. As she makes such sharing a consistent part of her interactions, Ted learns what her hands represent and the possibility of friendship. Dialogue surges above the trauma of the moment and translates the emerging relationship into expressions that eventually make sense to the other. As his fists are flying, we might say, "That is all right. I know you are afraid. I am not going to hurt you." These words need to be part and parcel of all our other interactions at the moment. And as we say these, we need to expand the dialogue so that the person learns, "When I am nervous, this caregiver is my friend." This helps develop a morality between the two that eventually flows outward.

The themes can emerge from the person's reality or our own. Even those interactions that symbolize marginalization bear much

Our first experiences involve
- Reflecting on themes for dialogue
- Developing them with creativity and imagination
- Concentrating on those that signify empathy and mutuality with the person within the person's reality
- Expressing them in words and other actions that convey authenticity
- Tolerating initial nonacceptance

fruit in relation to dialogue. While recognizing reality, we can give hope where there is despair. In Ted's case, it was the meaning of home. It varies from moment to moment and person to person.

John is a young man with schizophrenia. He sits in his classroom and slaps his raw ears. White pus and blood cover his shirt collar. He can hardly talk. His eyes rarely glance toward his teacher. When she asks him to do a task, he hits his ears several times and then wraps his hands and arms inside his shirt. The teacher sits beside him and quietly pushes away his school work. She takes one item so that she can try to encourage some participation, but focuses her attention on dialogue. What can she say? What can she do?

She works on the project with him, actually doing almost all of it, only lightly touching a piece of the task to his self-restrained hand. But as she does this she dialogues, "John, your eyes are so sad. Your heart is as if frozen over." She taps his chest playfully. "We have to thaw you out and watch the warm blood flow up to your face!" She goes on like this for several minutes. John's hands start to reach out slowly. He looks at her; a faint smile forms. These are the seedlings of dialogue.

When the person is withdrawn, self-injurious, or aggressive, the hunger for union is omnipresent, but secreted in the depths of the heart. We have to understand that, even though rejecting us, the person still longs for companionship and friendship. John's self-restrained arms and injured ears speak a multitude of feelings about himself, ourselves, and his world. Our hope is that one day soon his arms will reach toward us, his eyes will gaze upon us, and he will call us "friend." We need to grasp that the person's rejection emanates from a social history that defines us more as instruments of oppression in the institutional role of carrying out mechanistic "individualized plans" than as companions expressing a helping relationship.

In the example of "going home" or the "frozen heart," the themes are manifold: the possible meaning of home, its reality, the concept of homelessness, and the feeling of friendship. We need to ready ourselves to communicate these thoughts and feelings. This requires placing ourself in the other's reality and then conveying this to the person. Dialogue involves an on-going critical questioning of social reality and involves helping the other feel oneness with us and others. It should not avoid truth, but seek it out and express it.

The language itself should be as concrete and reality-based as possible. Yet it needs to deal with abstractions such as loneliness, anger, longings, and friendship. These can be expressed clearly through storytelling and allegories that relate to the person's life condition. Our feelings should convey a coming together. Dialogue is serious and playful, quiet and animated, as well as pensive and reflective. It is a balance of life's processes. And we are the ones who need to initiate it.

Eliciting and Expanding Dialogue

Eliciting dialogue is critical since without a mutual flow of communication it does not exist. Yet it does not have to be in words. Its center is the expression of feelings. One way to facilitate its reciprocation is to initiate it within a context of doing an activity together, since the task at hand can serve as a vehicle for structuring the interactions. While interacting, we have a structure to keep the engagement going and, while hands are busy, to center the interactions on dialogue and its elicitation.

Dialogue revolves around the expression of a feeling of being with and for the person, moving us from a role of staff to active

---

Eliciting Dialogue

- Recognize that the first encounters will be laborious
- Connect the dialogue with participation since it is structured
- Establish a soothing and warm tone and pace
- Look for any subtle responses and carefully elicit them
- Value any and all movements toward any reciprocation

---

participant with the person. The task gives us a structure to carry on what will initially be one-sided dialogue. This structure is especially helpful when initiating a dialogue with someone with severe behavioral problems, few communication skills, or little vocabulary. It provides a focus for us, if nothing else. Although the person will often be moving away, trying to attack you, trying to hurt self, or totally withdrawn, both the participation and dialogue should continue in spite of these acts of rejection. While mobilizing the best of our own personality, we need to concentrate on soothingness, nurturing, and guiding the person through the dialogue. We should not expect any initial response except passive participation, but we need to persevere since the ongoing giving of value and expression of dialogue leads to the eventual internalization of its meaning. In the beginning, we need to draw it out of the person, whether through concrete acts such as asking "Where's your smile?" or through more subtle elicitation such as the person allowing us to place our hand on theirs.

In this process, the person slowly begins to become linked with this spirit of dialogue. Whether cognitively understanding what is transpiring or not, the person starts to sense the warmth and begins to communicate attentiveness, serenity, and mutuality through gazes, smiles, and other forms of reaching out. Each speaks his or her own language, whether through words, sounds, or gestures. This might involve soothing vocalizations in someone who has been accustomed to screaming or crying spells. It might involve thumb-sucking in someone who has only been used to slamming their fists into walls. It might involve gently rocking to and fro for a person who has ordinarily only been tied up. It might involve a homeless person's sitting with us and reflecting on a personal view of life. It might involve a conversation, story-telling, listening, playful banter, teasing, or serious sharing about who we are and why we are together, as well as what we are doing and why we are doing it.

Let us recall John—the young man with schizophrenia—sitting before us—his shirt bloodied from self-injury, his head downcast, his eyes closed, his hands clasped together inside his shirt, his interest totally turned inward. He sees no meaning in us, nor in participation with us, nor in our valuing. How can we dialogue with him? He is supposedly nonresponsive and too disturbed to become involved in shared feelings.

As he sits rubbing his chafed ears against his shoulders, we place our hand on his shoulder to protect and soothe him. Then, with our other hand, we place a piece of a game on top of his hand, knowing it has little or no significance. After all, it is only a piece of plastic. Persevering and helping him in a warm and valuing way, we begin to gradually effectuate an ebb and flow of participation and separation from fear. He begins to feel slightly safe and secure. He starts to realize that our words are for valuing, not for demands or ridicule.

As we do this, we initiate our first dialogue. Its content is based on the concept that "I know that you feel wounded, but it is good to be together. I am not going to hurt you. We can learn to be friends." As time goes on, he begins to participate more and appears more attentive. When asked, "Are we friends?" he shakes his head "No!" But we continue.

In order to solidify the dialogue, we touch his "heart" and say, "Do you know what hearts are for?" and go on saying, "They are for warmth, and yours, like mine, is often cold, even frozen. But friendship melts the ice in our hearts." As we say this, we place our finger near his frowning mouth and say, "The melting water flows from our heart to our mouth and this is what makes us smile." This playful, yet serious, process continues. His dialogue is his allowing us to be closer to him, to touch him, and to be warm toward him.

Gradually, almost imperceptibly, he begins to gaze, smile, and quietly say, "Friend!" With this beginning, the caregiver expands the dialogue and incorporates his words or deeds into this growing feeling of companionship. It is a process that blossoms. Having nothing to do with chattering, it is a fusion of sharing with respect and warmth through our words, gestures, and physical interactions.

Those who can speak and understand are more readily seen as capable of entering into a dialogue. Yet words are not the key. The center rests on emotional expressions. Some might say that a person with severe mental retardation or acute mental illness is unable to communicate, and, thus, dialogue is impossible. Or they might say that John cannot understand abstractions such as friendship, the meaning of sharing, or the inherent goodness of human engagement. Indeed, John might not be able to categorize these conditions; but he is a sentient being and is touched by the quality of life's experiences, both those that have beaten him down and those that now seek to lift him up. Dialogue is a central part of the human condition. Its expression, breadth, and depth evolve over time. Each person expresses self and dialogues according to different modalities and intensities, moving from almost imperceptible signs to complex communication. The vital aspect for us is to be sensitive to these varying and unfolding forms, be reflective of these feelings with empathy and acceptance, and be open to the communicative nature of the person's interactions. We become more naturally warm when a give-and-take develops. We begin to

---

Dialogue's expansion involves
- Deepening warmth and genuine regard
- Weaving together seriousness and playfulness
- Increasingly personalizing the tone and content
- Eliciting feelings—at first minute expressions, then ever-growing ones
- Reaching more deeply into the other's life condition
- Increasing warm interactions with the person

sense the person's here-and-now mood and modulate our tone. And, in due course, we bring others into the dialogue as a means of sharing and expanding an evolving circle of friends.

Dialogue makes the coming together of the caregiver and the marginalized person a concrete expression of the human condition based on justice. Life does not exist without others. In effect it says, "You and I are one." The relationship slowly evolves and expands outward. We cannot reach out to others if we do not continually question who we are and how we exist in relation to others. This has to occur in relation to our whole reality. We have to ask ourselves and others why we are engaged in work among the marginalized and define it in the light of mutual liberation. We need to see, feel, and practice this relationship in our daily lives. We cannot reach out and signal union to the other if we do not recognize our own interdependence. And those on the fringe of society will never accept our presence, nor participate with us, nor value themselves or us if we do not enter into a spirit of dialogue with them. The development of a spirit of dialogue toward marginalized persons involves a lifetime of struggle and commitment.

The evolving purpose of this coming together is to establish a collective of companions in which community can form. This small group develops into a growing circle of friends. Schools slowly become places of learning solidarity and sharing, where the strong help the weak and the fast accompany the slow. Teachers need to give an example of friendship and teach the children to help each other. Traditional learning is important, but secondary. Indeed, it is enhanced by emotional connectedness, and it expands the more the child or adult feels one with the world. The driving force in the classroom becomes the teaching of human solidarity. This occurs in simple ways: doing projects together, helping the children reach out to one another; taking recess in groups; translating reading, writing, and arithmetic into the surrounding reality. Those who work with the institutionalized begin to focus on developing self-advocacy and establishing programs and services that are run by the people themselves. Incarcerated people are helped to organize and speak for themselves, while together we help to fight for their rights by supporting the creation of integrated communities. Programs become much more than facilities; they start to reflect companionship, justice, and social change. Group home workers' primary challenge is to create a home—not a building made of bricks, but one constructed with love and affection in which a sense of family is created. Parents struggle to bring their difficult child into the warm embrace of the family, school, and neighborhood. It is through these transformations of purposes that we can bring about deepened community where the marginalized are with us at the center.

Regardless of diagnoses, and in spite of total rejection, we take the initial step in the development of a dialogue. This begins with the full acceptance and affirmation of the mind–body–spirit–emotional totality of the other. Our initiation of dialogue is at the core of the emerging feeling of companionship. It is the blood that runs in the veins of caregiving. It links us together and creates a process of widening union.

Our words are actually secondary. Dialogue is not mere conversation, nor can it be solely analyzed as a flow of words in a stimulus-response cycle. It is the feelings we convey, the warmth of our expression, and the sense of a coming together; it is a give-and-take, but within the context of these feelings. Essentially, we turn toward the other and share the moment to moment reality in all things serious and trivial. We recognize that all persons have the strength and potential for the expression of union. This depends upon the expression of sentiments, no matter how imperceptible, such as smiles, gazes, the giving and receiving of value, and any other signs of oneness.

> Kevin is a young man with severe depression. He has lost his speech, his self-care skills, and his desire to participate due to the death of his mother and father and his subsequent loss of life meaning and solidarity. He sees himself as alone and floundering. He feels that there is no one who can rescue him. He spends his days seated in a foster home, nearly catatonic and motionless. His caregivers are totally perplexed and fearful that he is on the brink of death.

Then one day his foster mother decides to focus on the creation of friendship. She realizes that she has to recreate a feeling of
being with others to instill hope where despair now reigns. But
what do you say to a nearly catatonic person? She reflects on the
fact that Kevin is like her own son and thinks about what stories she
tells her own children. That evening she brings a book and reads
it to him. It is a story about how a parent loves her child and cares
for him, and, as the years pass, how the child, now grown, cares for
his loving parent. As she tells it, she affectionately holds his
clenched hands. Every few moments she lovingly repeats this re-
frain, "I'll love you forever; I'll like you for always. As long as I am
living, my friend you will be." The first few times seem to mean
nothing to Kevin. Then he occasionally glances at her. Soon, a faint
smile emerges on his face. And then, almost inaudibly, he begins to
repeat, "I'll love you forever; I'll like you for always. As long as I am
living, my friend you will be." These halting words fall from his
faintly smiling face like the sun breaking through dark clouds. This
is only the beginning of a new life for Kevin based on the hope of
being one with others—but he is off to a good start.

Dialogue is based on a clear expression of the self in relation
to the other. It is an ongoing expression of feelings. These ema-
nate from the inner person and are seen in movement toward the
other. It is not only a turning of the body toward the other, but
more basically a turning of the spirit in an affirmation of the
other's being and a reflecting of the other in ourselves. Kevin's
foster mother was willing to give of herself by sharing an intimate
part of her own life.

RELATIONSHIPS BASED ON DIALOGUE

This self-surrendering starts from the moment we are con-
ceived. The mother bears the child and gives love and affection.
This nurturing is embraced by the family. As dependent as the
infant is, giving is made concrete in the mother's feeding, cud-
dling, bathing, and singing. These expressions transcend words
and are freely given. They are dialogue. They require a surrender

of self, but also a self-fulfillment. The baby smiles, coos, and reaches out. These are signs of dialogue and love. The message is life-giving. The act of loving the other gives life to the one loving as well as to the beloved. To speak words of love and to show signs and symbols of affection is to be loved as well as to love. Dialogue signifies a coming together. It is the convergence of human beings with one another in a spirit of solidarity. It means a reflection of our equality—not sameness, but oneness. It means giving—not giving up, but giving of oneself.

Outside of the almost naturally unfolding mother–infant bond, caregivers come face-to-face with persons who have no bonded relationships. For any number of reasons, these represent bonds never fully developed, never expanded beyond the family, or bonds that were severed. Or limited relationships exist, but are not strong enough to go beyond a small circle. And when that network disappears, the person is left helpless and vulnerable. Some might feel that dialogue under these conditions is impossible and an exercise in futility and that control is the only option. However, caring means our recognition and full awareness of the inherent value of the other person. It means caring about, not just caring for, the other. It is a process of surrender based on our recognition that the other person, regardless of needs, is deserving of respect and is seen in his or her human wholeness. Giving care is not the mere act of caring for bodily needs or dealing with disorganized behaviors. We need to recognize that giving is a process that embraces our own potentialities and fulfillment—with the greatest gift being the act of giving self to the other. Although caregiving might involve taking care of bodily needs, it more acutely signifies caring enough to enter into and engender a spirit of interdependence and solidarity with others. This is uniquely different from paternalistic or materialistic acts since it is based on equality and an ever-growing coming together. This synthesis is a fundamental assumption in caregiving centered on dialogue. In essence, we commit ourselves to nurture-bonded relationships, and dialogue is the thread that weaves this together.

Respect for the "least among us" can be clearly seen among

those who give care to persons with the severest dimensions of mental retardation, AIDS babies, the acutely mentally ill, and other ostracized persons. Caregivers who serve those who cannot speak, walk, or care for themselves affirm the fullness of the other in spite of these tremendous needs. As these caregivers help clean and give nourishment, they simultaneously see themselves in these dependent persons and conclude that all are dependent upon one another. This respect helps to give rise to dialogue. The bedridden child or adult who cannot speak communicates through gazes and slight movements. The act of caregiving itself can be a dialogue.

Parents and other caregivers who are shocked, frustrated, or insulted by rejection and distancing need to regroup, re-examine their interactions, and move toward the expression and elicitation of valuing and dialogue. This requires much energy and a turning away from the modern-day tendency to view desired change as a process of being shaped to comply to external power. Interdependence implies something quite different. Teams of professionals often meet to discuss the needs of "patients" or "clients" in order to delineate programs based on reward or punishment to achieve compliance. This might be effective if compliance is the goal. However, we all need much more than these efficient, externalized behavioral approaches. This type of shallow searching for manageable solutions inevitably misses the point that people need to be totally accepted as they are and in spite of their distancing behavior. Behavior problems will evaporate like the morning dew if we express unconditional valuing. Thus, although their behaviors can be objectively termed as acts of aggression or self-injury that need to be controlled through the dual behavioral system of reward and punishment, such control proves to be meaningless and sterile. Dialogue is our option. It does not see the individual as a lesser being. It reaches out, not down. It uplifts us as well as the person. While recognizing marginalization and emotional apartness, dialogue embraces companionship as a sign of union, as opposed to compliance and force.

Violence leads to violence, restraint to restraint. The logic of control has a bottomless tool box. However, change is based on more than what is seen and quantifiable; it goes beyond psychological arithmetic and, indeed, calls for the exploration and definition of both inner anguish and joy. It requires us to feel the human condition, help heal anguish, and share in hopefulness. It leads us to see what is unseen, hear what is unspoken, and feel what is often unfelt through empathy. It brings us to the threshold of understanding the signs and symbols of the other person. Although the most disconnected person may not speak, hear, walk, or move, we need to arrive at a point in which we can dialogue with the voiceless person. It is this giving that transforms apartness into union.

A Leap of Faith

The final characteristic in a relationship based on dialogue is the most difficult; yet, once accepted, it is the warmest and most expressive of authenticity. Caregiving requires a leap of faith in the recognition and acceptance of the wholeness of the other and the interdependence of the other with us. It asks us to believe that unconditional acceptance and valuing is central to significant behavioral change. This leap can be most paradoxical. When we are confronted with persons who are hitting, biting, kicking, and scratching, we are asked to see the other's worth and find ways to respect and uplift the other in spite of violent reactions. Violence can bring out the worst in us or the best. As spit rolls down our face, the question of embracing the wholeness of the other is necessarily fragile. As fingernails dig into our skin, a common reaction is to become forceful. Yet, while preventing such acts as much as possible, we still must position ourselves to give value, in spite of whatever is transpiring, and reach into ourselves to continue to value the other. Dialogue is the highest expression of this valuing and the deepest affirmation of the wholeness of both ourselves and the other.

CONCLUSION

In essence, we make a choice between monologue and dialogue and between interactions based on contingency and those
centered on giving value. Monologue implies an entirely different
posture. It establishes compliance and control as the major rationale for our intervention. It embraces reward or punishment as the
means to achieve these ends. It sees everyone's fulfillment as independence with each responsible for self-survival and self-regu-
lation. It replaces a feeling of union with an objectifiable state of
behavioral management. It centers itself on deeds done rather
than the centrality of being with the other. On the other hand,
dialogue accepts the other in spite of acts of violence. It gives value
to the person regardless of deeds done. It is not interested in
reward or punishment, but in respecting and valuing the person.
It is at the very heart of a feeling of companionship. Its words and
expressions are like the flow of warm blood that gives life. It is an
act of justice and solidarity.

Chapter 6
TESTIMONIALS TO DIALOGUE

Since dialogue is so deeply rooted in our own values and our perceptions of the worth of marginalized individuals, it is critical that we understand the total commitment that such genuine openness requires. Dialogue calls on us to recognize our own and the other person's reality, to judge the way that we can open ourselves to him or her, and then enter into a process that leads to the establishment of feelings of companionship.

In recent years, we have encountered thousands of marginalized persons and have learned from them. Initial conditions have been horrendous: We have seen people locked up, tied up, homeless, drugged, and beaten. Those whom we see and work among are often voiceless, and, even if they can speak, words cannot describe their encompassing and seething hopelessness. Yet their full humanity calls on us. We ask, "Why is she slamming her head on the floor? Why is he being shoved into a padded room? Why are those children living on top of a garbage dump among pigs and flies? Why has this parent given up?" To give care is to deepen and instill hope; but such realities can leave us blind and cynical. If this occurs, despair soon follows. Fortunately, hope can be seen in those who move deeply into the process of companionship, even in the midst of oppression.

In the following testimonials, each person can provide us with insight that change is possible, if we are willing to be open to it and struggle for it. In these real-life examples, the major part of the struggle was to find ways to express dialogue.

113

ANNE

Some people are erroneously said to be beyond the reach of human reward, valuing, and dialogue. Some hold that the best that can be expected is to gain control over these persons' behaviors. Yet we assume that valuing and dialogue are possible and can become meaningful. Even when the person flails, hits, and kicks, our driving force is to unconditionally value the person through dialogue. This expression takes root in the other the more we give it. As confusion swirls around, we continue. As we behold the oppressed, we deepen our valuing. As we take the hand's sting to our face, we go on.

Anne sat alone. She was tied to a chair in the corridor of a locked ward in a public institution for the mentally ill. She was clearly being kept apart from all others. Her caregivers were more like guards than companions, more like jail keepers than friends. Her face was vacant except for a pained expression: Her eyes were cast downward, and her lips were curled in anger and hatred. She occasionally looked at those passing by her, but this was only to ensure that no one approached her. Fear was mutual. She was ready to scream or slam her head into any hard surface to drive others away from her. She lived a life of monologue in a culture of death. She mumbled to herself, "Hate! Hate! Hate!" No one paid attention to her words. She was considered a non-person. Her head and arms were marked with sores, scratches, and contusions—from her own self-beatings and aggression by others. Each pockmark spoke stories of despair, solitude, and marginalization. She sat "embraced" by the leather straps bolted to her wooden chair. She was like the queen of loneliness, with embracing arms replaced by straps and a wooden chair for a throne. Her crown was a masked helmet. In her kingdom, there was no joy, only despair; no otherness, only aloneness; no relatedness, only empty existence; no dialogue, only monologue.

Her life consisted of being controlled by others, and her subsequent violent reactions were meant to control her controllers. Treatment involved encountering violence with violence. Of course, she was outnumbered by caretakers, and they won every battle. They charted her every move. Their monologue was enunciated, not by words, but by acts of submission. Their hands pulled her into the chair and tightened the straps. Their faces spoke of their dislike of her and her absurd world. Their footsteps echoed their separation from her and signalled that they were only available for her management. She sat alone, "comforted" only by leather and wood. Her fleeting looks and her muted moans spoke of fear. Her forlorn countenance spoke of a history of isolation and rejection, but hinted at a longing for otherness. Occasionally, she would glance at someone as if hoping for something more. But dialogue could not occur since there were no others in union with her.

Many reasons were given for the "need" for restraint. Her head banging was "life-threatening," and restraint was "the only option." Indeed, one day her psychologist discovered the latest device, an automated electric shock instrument. This, he proclaimed, once connected to her body, would end the self-injury and the need for life-long restraint. The caretaking monologue evolved like sounds delivered between parallel people with no convergence. Its syntax was represented by control, and an electric shock device was the latest symbol of this soliloquy. Its current of pain, if strong enough, would terminate her self-injury.

Then, one day, due to public pressure and horror related to the recommended use of an instrument of torture such as the shock device, even in the name of treatment, she was ordered released from her wooden throne and its straps and was placed in a setting where her caregivers decided to teach her to feel secure, participate, and valued. In their first attempts, she demanded, "My helmet!" She knew that she was driven by fear and that freedom would result in injury. "My helmet!" she cried over and over again. Her face was angry. Her fists pounded the caregivers.

But this process was to be different: No restraint and no punishment. It was to be based on their expression of solidarity with her, even though she had no sentiments for this, no feeling of union, and was totally apart from the flow of human interdependence. The first step in the creation of a spirit of dialogue with a person accustomed to monologue is to give an outpouring of valuing while at the same time replacing old meanings; all those interactions that were devaluing, distancing, and disconnecting have to be emptied of their power.

In Anne's case, this meant that she had to be protected, but not restrained. For a few hours, two caregivers had to be with her. They had to become accustomed to the speed with which she injured herself and learn to make her safe. She had to get an inkling that they would not hurt her. Every movement had to signal valuing. Every action had to be instantaneously looked at from an interactional perspective. Every contact had to answer the question, "Does this help transmit a feeling of valuing, warmth, and nurturing?"—each caregiver's expression had to transmit these feelings. Their hands had to represent valuing rather than oppression and domination. Their words had to signal authenticity and genuineness. These actions had to be given with no expectation of any reciprocation, but always with hope for it. Dialogue had to be entered into with tolerance, with little expectation of any immediate reply, and with ardor. It had to be communicated with hope, even though initially it was known that their presence meant nothing to her.

At first, she responded with anger and violence: She slapped a caregiver in the face, pulled her hair, and retreated from any physical approximations. She kept begging for her helmet since it was her symbol for controlling the jail-like world in which she had lived. Restraint had become the center of her life and no person was going to replace this meaning, as absurd as it might have been. In spite of this, her caregivers persevered. They had to be ready to accept her no matter what. They had to be ready to be attacked and still give value while protecting themselves.

As they continued to immerse themselves into giving value, Anne slowly and occasionally began to come closer to them. Once in a while she looked at the caregivers, reached out, and eventually even showed the faintest flicker of a smile. Of course, these moments were few in the beginning. Most of the time was spent protecting her from self-injury and attempting to bring about engagement. Nevertheless, the flickering signs of dialogue had started, and she had started to accept these caregivers and then others who had been observing.

On her own, Anne began to glance playfully at them. As this began to unfold, her attempts at self-injury slowly started to disappear when she was with them. Their presence was taking on a new meaning. The original value-giving was converting itself into a warm conversation in the form of songs, story-telling, and a spirit of playfulness. The caregivers had to be cautious not to value her only when she was doing whatever she was supposed to be doing. The focus had to be on their emerging relationship. Since modern practices tend to be relegated to the realm of reward for deeds done, it was critical that they rupture this practice by giving value for her human condition rather than her achievements. Valuing-transforming-itself-into-dialogue had to be given regardless of her replies.

Soon the flickering smile exploded into laughter. Individual caregivers started to be with her on their own. She began to curiously reach out to the first two and then the other caregivers. She started to sing with them and invent songs with them. After three days of increasing dialogue, she broke out into a joyous smile on one occasion and said, "I am going to go home someday!"

At the start, the caregivers had to protect Anne. However, by the time of her first smile, they were able to use their hands for giving value rather than protection. Their interactions began to take on a more playful and joyful meaning. What had been driven and impulsive was now slowing down into a peaceful rhythm, best symbolized by a calm rocking that she would do when with these caregivers. She also began to embrace them. Since trust, safety, and security were now emerging, she was content to be engaged with one or the other of these caregivers. They were able to be less intense and "on guard" against self-injury. Friendliness replaced protection, and joking substituted for screaming and moaning. The interactions were taking on the meaning of companionship.

As this happened, she also became open to more complex change and the introduction of new persons into her life, including persons whom she had previously been kept away from "due to her severe behaviors." She began to play cards and enjoy other activities. She became interested in giving value to others rather than just receiving it. Her sweet "bye-byes" at the end of each day signalled the beginning of a spirit of sharing and bonded relationships. The burning electricity of the recommended cattle prod had been replaced by human warmth.

Thus unfolds the process of a relationship based on dialogue between caregivers and a distanced person. This needs to continue throughout Anne's life or it will wither and die, just as in our own lives. Few words were ever spoken by Anne, yet she was quite capable of expressing her inner self and her emerging union with her caregivers. She became able to elicit strong feelings of joy in those around her with her warming movements. She and her caregivers began to signify solidarity and interdependence. The delicate lace that held this fabric together was dialogue.

SHAWN

Another example of this process is that of a young man named Shawn. He lived in a group home with four other devalued men. He spent most of his days locked in a seclusion room next to the kitchen. He was big, strong, and aggressive. His psychiatrist had solemnly concluded that his mental retardation and organic brain syndrome were the causes of his hopeless aggression. The center of his life had become the seclusion room. Like Anne Marie, he begged for restraint. His only intelligible words were, "Time out! Time out! Time out!" Almost anytime he was asked, or more typically ordered, to do a task or activity, he demanded to be placed in seclusion. If this demand did not work, he would then dig his fingers into his rectum and show his soiled fingers to his caregivers and repeat, "Time out!" If one did not "escort" him to this place of solitude, he would continue his ritual with each caregiver until someone would finally lock him in the room. He preferred the exile of the time-out room to the domination and frigidity of his caretakers. He also attacked them or fellow residents who got in the way of his seclusion. He would open his mouth in anger and dig his teeth into their hands or arms. His life of monologue was quite controlling and reflected the world in which he lived, wherein solitude had become preferable to participation and caregivers had opted to become jailers.

In his caregivers' first feeble attempt to teach Shawn to live in harmony with them, he reacted violently. They were cynical toward the idea of unconditional valuing. He sensed their phoniness. They did not dialogue, their words to him were few and depended on his compliance. They had to begin to change their beliefs and practices. When Shawn saw them, he stood up and went to each with his left hand digging into his rectum, and yelled, almost chanting, "Time out!" He bounced off each of them like a pinball as they stood with their arms crossed and their heads nodding to "get back to work." Unfortunately, for them, this was "dialogue." Finally, in exasperation, he attacked a caregiver. His wide open mouth moved rapidly into flesh and his hatred was confirmed in this mix of teeth and skin. His caregivers were not prepared to value or engage him.

Before they could begin the process, they had to question themselves, their values, and how to express dialogue. They had to reflect on what their posture was and whether they wanted to convey this spirit or simply subdue him. This took time and debate. They looked at themselves and examined their own actions. Slowly, they resolved to choose companionship. They decided that it was important to connect valuing with participation since he was not only aggressive but also self-isolating. They began to realize that they had to dramatically increase and intensify their unconditional valuing and bring about any approximation toward any engagement with them. They finally knew they needed to help him to engage in participatory interactions as a means of creating a new interactional context, even though one caregiver insisted that Shawn was manipulating them for attention saying, "He knows better. He is just tricking you!" However, the others chose to try to persevere and center all their interactions on valuing.

On subsequent occasions when he tried to bite, they continued to give him value and enable participation while simultaneously protecting themselves. They spoke of friendship and how it was important and good to be with him. This required much diligence since they were teaching one another how to give unconditional valuing. When he started to yell "time out," they told him that they would take a break together. All their words began to concentrate on the goodness of being with him. Slowly, instead of hitting, he would stop his arm in mid-air, look in a puzzled manner at the particular caregiver, close his mouth, and engage in the particular activity. This afforded the caregivers the opportunity to express valuing more intensely and increase his participatory interactions.

These moments were the seedlings of dialogue. The fact that he reconsidered his actions in midstream meant that he was beginning to reflect on the possibility of union and was beginning to view these caregivers not as jail keepers, but as other human beings with the potential for being trusted.

As the next days unfolded, Shawn became more accepting of valuing and his caregivers became more authentic and genuine. He began to reciprocate it in the form of kissing their hands instead of biting them, patting their heads instead of hitting, and shaking their hands instead of digging into his rectum. As this began to transpire, his acts of violence also started to diminish in frequency and intensity, and he became involved in a range of tasks and activities for long periods of time. This young man, who had only expressed the sad vocabulary of isolation, soon started to whisper words of warm and contented feelings to these caregivers. These were accompanied by smiles and moving his caregivers' hands to his chest and smiling peacefully. This, then, is what dialogue was for Shawn: emerging signs and symbols of friendship, companionship, and sentiments of union. It was the confirmation of his self in relation to his caregivers. And what about the seclusion room? It was made into a closet and Shawn never chanted "time out" again.

ROSA

Rosa was a 4-year-old girl who was born without any complications. But when she was 9 months old a metal shelf fell on her head and caused severe brain damage resulting in paralysis on her right side, loss of speech, and the appearance of self-injurious behaviors in the form of rapidly moving her left hand into her mouth and biting it forcefully. As she had not been restrained, this behavior had resulted in her yanking out her fingernails. But in spite of these challenges and the fact that she was eventually put in restraint, her mother and father nurtured her at home. They gave her warmth and uncalculated affection. She attended a regular kindergarten class and participated in family activities. Yet the burden was great. Having searched for an answer to the self-injury and having found none, her parents placed her left arm in restraint and continued to integrate her into the family.

Rosa was quite obviously a loved and loving child. Yet she continued to engage in this self-harm whenever free from the plastic restraint tube on her arm. Ironically, she was quick to smile and be affectionate in her interactions. However, once released from restraint, she inevitably attempted to bite herself. Her tiny hand moved with lightening speed to mouth. As the months passed, she became less integrated with her family and less likely to live a life of union with others since the self-injury and restraint were gradually replacing her natural warmth and frustrating her parents. The restraint, as necessary as it was, had started to become the center of her parent's relationship with her. The necessary protection was suffocating the child's being since it favored apartness over union. The arm tube had become more important than reaching out. Her mother was saddened by her decreasing participation and an increasing need to subdue her for the sake of avoiding harm.

> Rosa's re-entrance into the fullness of human dialogue with others began with the assurance that no harm would come to her, and she was loosened from her restraint. Her parents were rightfully worried about her safety. In the first hours, her mother sat with her and used her own arms and hands to "shadow" the child's attempts at self-harm, hovering one hand above the child's to block any attempted bites. While doing this, she worked hand-over-hand with her on various games and used this as the way to express warm and playful valuing. She told her stories about her two older brothers, and talked to her about how beautiful she was. Rosa listened intently and made a few sounds of delight. Yet, if her mother were to remove her hand for a split second, Rosa would immediately try to bite herself and yank out her fingernails. It was difficult to block these attempts. In the first few hours, the mother grabbed her daughter's hand almost automatically; yet with practice she learned to protect rather than restrain.

Rosa's mother began to elicit more valuing by expecting Rosa to get more involved in the stories. She asked her to identify play blocks as family members and she had Rosa kiss each one. She asked her, "Now you kiss mommy!" and helped her hug and kiss. Rosa was very happy to do this. She started to play more, smile, and nod her head. The mother gradually lifted her hand from Rosa's, but was still ready to shadow any dangerous movement, while also continuing the story and increasing physical, verbal, and gestural valuing. As the child became more engrossed in the stories, she attempted to bite herself less and gaze lovingly at her mother. This enabled her mother to protect her less and concentrate more on the dialogue. Other caregivers were introduced and all followed the same process.

After several days, the caregivers were able to avoid grasping Rosa's hand. By the fourth day, she began to move her finger to her tongue and indicate the desire for a kiss. The first time she did this, her mother feared that she was going to bite her finger, and much to her joy, she soon saw that it was her way of saying, "Kiss me!" Her little finger was now not for biting, but for pointing for a kiss. She became more engaged. What had been cries turned to humming songs. Her humming began to sound more like words.

Then one day her mother was playing her in a make-believe telephone conversation. Picking up the toy phone, she pretended to call Rosa. The child watched and smiled. The mother carried on a conversation, "How are you, Rosa?" The child shook her head playfully. The mother said, "I just called to say I love you!" Rosa smiled and her mother began to tell her about all the people who loved her. At the end of a few moments, the child was laughing. The mother slowly and warmly said, "Rosa, I . . . love . . . you . . ." She repeated the phrase and invited the child to say the same words. Surprisingly, Rosa, with all of her emotional and physical might, made sounds that approximated the phrase, "I . . . love . . you!" She was imitating the same cadence and intonation of her mother's dialogue. Each sound and word fell from her lips like rain drops on the parched earth. Affection gave birth to affection, sounds imitated sounds, and warmth replaced self-harm. The seedlings of dialogue were unearthed in this child's heart by her mother and teachers.

Conclusion

Through these three testimonials, we have set forth real life examples of the expression of dialogue among those who had been disenfranchised from it. All three individuals had been subjected to restraint or punishment. Yet all were able to enter into a process in which they began to express unconditional ongoing valuing. This validated their very humanness, encouraged them and their caregivers, and helped to transform all involved. They and their caregivers knew that they had stepped onto the edge of the life-long road toward a culture of life. They realized that this journey would be marked with fertile land, rather than with the desert of containment; it would be filled with hope generating surprises instead of the monotony of restraint and the isolation of helplessness; and, most importantly, it would be a journey done with others. It is this mystery of living life in solidarity that gives meaning to the human condition, and it is this grassroots daily engagement that brings about union. The caregivers' time and energy was significant. It was no easy task to spend hours and days tilling the soul of hope. It took the mastery of skills, the creativity of putting their values into action, and ongoing questioning and mutual support.

We have seen that dialogue does not depend upon words alone, although it is enhanced by them; basically, it arises out of a deep undercurrent of feelings on the bed of human commonality. Its waters join individuals together. Each has his or her own being, about to be connected by the ebb and flow of a bonded relationship. At the start, the caregiver is bolstered by the breeze of giving and the hope of transformation; the other is bent by the winds of marginalization. The caregiver bears the responsibility for entering into dialogue; the other has no evident reason to accompany the caregiver at the beginning of the journey, other than a hidden hope for interdependence. This is clouded by fear, repugnance, or confusion. It is the caregiver who must give meaning to the po-

tentially emergent relationship through respect, equality, and valuing in spite of strong initial rejection. Over time, this longing
surfaces, dialogue unfolds, and feelings of companionship start to
follow. Regardless of the severity of the marginalized condition—
whether founded on mental retardation, mental handicap, old
age, infirmity, racism, or poverty—it is assumed that dialogue is
possible. It is a process which begins with two distinct beings
coming together and becoming one in spirit. The one cares for the
well-being of the other and vice versa. Both are givers and each
becomes more in the process.

Chapter 7
THE PROCESS OF MUTUAL CHANGE

A psychology of interdependence brings us and marginalized persons into a mutual change process. Caregiving involves the recognition of an ongoing struggle in which we reject domination and opt for valuing. It asks us to define, center, and practice a process of unfolding solidarity. This, then, leads us to assume the responsibility for establishing new meanings in the human condition and rejecting old ones founded on control and domination. Solidarity arises from a view that both we and the other person hunger for feelings of relatedness and that our commitment to this initiates a mutual change process. However, nothing will solidify until we make the decision to become interdependent and reflect on how we can express this in our daily interactions.

Caregiving is an option to serve those who are marginalized: children, the mentally retarded, the mentally ill, the poor, the elderly, the disenfranchised, the homeless, and all persons kneeling on the floor of the community's banquet hall searching for the leftovers of our feast. Each of these individuals, once alienated, survives by his or her aggression, self-injury, or withdrawal. Their lives take on meaning through these behaviors, but a meaning that further pushes them away from others. We have seen how important our beliefs are and how companionship can be established through dialogue. We have examined the elements that undergo change in this process and have described these.

CHANGING MEANINGS

Yet the question remains: "What sequence of events will likely transpire in the establishment of new meanings in the relationship?" We go through a change process with each person. When the other is disharmonious, we need to express harmony. As the person begins to engage with us, we still need to expect the reappearance of rejection. Yet in time these moments become less intense and briefer. With our perseverance, a bonded relationship slowly forms. At this moment, we then need to help the person expand this feeling to others. The entire process involves a gradual putting aside of old meanings and learning new ones.

Our challenge is to generate a process that changes the meaning of the human condition. Alienation is worsened by our enchantment with self-reliance and obedience to social norms. Our view is that we were born neither to be independent, nor dependent; to be neither masters, nor peons. Although our culture exalts the "self-made" and "survivors," independence contradicts feelings of solidarity, democracy, and union. It places women and men in a state of solitude in which each lives parallel to the other. It means that each is apart from the other with no connections of any substance. It is essentially a materialistic perspective and one based on domination. It assumes that the primary purpose of life is to develop one's own skills and to use these for the benefit of self. The best for a few leads to something less for the many—often significantly and sorrowfully so.

Although there are persons who depend more on others for basic bodily or material needs, this does not imply that they are any less, nor have nothing to share. The humblest person can be the most insightful poet. The most mentally disorganized can possess the deepest spiritual feelings. The most mentally handicapped can bring the profoundest perception of being human. The aged can remind us of who we are and what we are becoming. The most hungry can teach us about our bounty and the meaning of justice. On the ridge between dependence and independence stands the strong and weak, the able and unable in a spirit of interdependence. This affirms our being and leads us into a process of becoming one with the other.

Interdependence makes caregiving an acutely conscious process wherein we do not seek to "normalize" behaviors or control them; rather, it is a one wherein we define our vocation as the unfolding of companionship, first within the dyad, then among others. It also recognizes that human valuing, although rooted in everyone's being, is initially meaningless since it has been buried beneath years of oppression. Our role is to bring it to the light of day. As we uncover this, what had been intolerable is tolerated; what had been destructive begins to disappear; what had been distancing becomes uniting; and what had been oppressive becomes centered on justice.

A MUTUAL PROCESS

Life is an ongoing process that involves constant change, and our deeds and interactions are based on what we believe, whether we are conscious of this or not. If we believe that we were born to rule over others, then our caregiving will center on this. If we believe that we exist to produce, then we will make our decisions based on that. If we believe that we are all brothers and sisters, then we will strive to create just communities. We have a marked tendency to dominate over the weak, and it is an ongoing struggle to change this, especially when confronted with violence. The moment someone threatens us, we want to retaliate; or, when someone refuses to do what we want, we are driven to modify that noncompliance. We need to transform our own interactions in a deliberate and conscious manner. Just as we have to facilitate a change process in the other, so, too, we need to undergo the same process ourselves. Change, then, is mutual. But the question still gnaws at us: "How can I establish a spirit of companionship?" Or more specifically, "What do I do when John is throwing the dishes on the floor? When Maria is having a tantrum? Or when Ted is ripping off his shirt? Or when Shawn is biting me?" The answer always swings back to unconditional valuing, at the best of times and the worst of times.

The creation of companionship and community never arrives at a "final" product. It deepens and expands, but does not end. It is an unfolding rather than a distinct end in itself. However, there are benchmarks in decreasing aggression, self-injury, and withdrawal, and increasing participation and decreasing fear on our

The Mutual Process

Caregiver	Dimension	Person
Opting for a culture of life Initiation of new meanings	Disharmony ↓	Rejection and avoidance Expression of anguish and apartness through aggression, self-injury, or withdrawal
Increasing capacity to prevent problems, to enable participation, and personalize dialogue Occasional, but increasing, elicitation of valuing	Intermittent acceptance ↓	Occasional, but increasing, acceptance of valuing Ebb and flow of engagement Some reciprocation of valuing
The giving and elicitation of unconditional valuing in increasingly natural ways	Bonding and companionship ↓	Gradual internalization of the meaning of human presence, engagement, and valuing The acceptance and reciprocation of unconditional valuing in increasingly natural ways
The extension of friendship to others The establishment of a spirit of union in homes, classrooms, and work places	Interdependence	The acceptance of sharing with others The integration of self into the fullness of community and family life

part and on the other's. It is not a lock-step process; rather, it involves an ebb and flow with good moments gradually overtaking difficult ones. The initial relationship gradually expands and becomes an integral part of our culture at school, work, and home. But it starts in a dimension of disharmony before it moves toward interdependence.

We move through various dimensions of change along with the person served. In essence, the process is comprised of distancing interactions losing their meaning as we establish a new meaning for coming together. Both might initially feel disharmony, but, as caregivers, we have to opt for a culture of life, ensure safety and security, and promote valuing and participation by designifying the meaning of aggression, self-injury, or withdrawal while resignifying companionship as the center of the human condition. The person's disharmony gradually unfolds into an on-again, off-again harmony. We need to understand that there will be an ebb and flow, but that valuing and its reciprocation will slowly become more meaningful. As this occurs, feelings of companionship begin to emerge and eventually expand outward to others, if we enable and facilitate it. It is within this process, context, and spirit that ongoing change occurs.

Harmony–Disharmony

Disharmony exists when a person sees no value in the other, finds no reason to be in union, nor feels any meaning in being valued by or valuing that person. It exemplifies itself in rage toward others or self. It is a movement away from humanizing contact. It signifies an inner turmoil, a disconnectedness, and even disgust with self and others. It can exist in anyone at anytime. It is not solely the burden of the dispossessed. Caregivers who seek to overpower the powerless, control the weak, or separate the humble are as disharmonious as the subjugated. We have a responsibility to be harmonious in the face of this disharmony, to check our fears and intolerance, and to center ourselves on valuing.

We need to question our purposes and our methods, especially during the most turbulent moments. For example, when a
person lashes out, what purpose does seclusion serve? Does it
protect him or control him? When a person cowers in fear and a
caregiver demands compliance, is this helping her or controlling
her? Often, we do not realize the impact of our actions, even
relatively insignificant ones.

Persons already in a state of disharmony do not require much
to signal that a particular caregiver or setting is oppressive and
dominative: keys hanging from belt loops, locked doors, posted
rules, disdainful gestures, mockery, rigid schedules, depersonalized interactions, condescending conversations, tokens, time-out
rooms, seclusion rooms, uniforms for caregivers (to distinguish
them from the marginalized), rights given as privileges, and a host
of other symbols. The caregiver who yells and orders others
around, who demands compliance, and who distributes rewards
or punishments like a landowner overseeing field hands clearly
communicates a disharmony within self, an insecurity, and a need
to dominate. The parent who yells and swats the child is crying, "I
do not know what to do. What will bring my child to me!" The
teacher who focuses on skill acquisition over engagement or who
interacts with the person only for deeds done clearly communicates this same feeling. The psychologist who uses punishment in
the name of therapy symbolizes a dominative value system that, in
fact, only reflects an inner drive to overpower the powerless. The
volunteer cook in the soup kitchen who forbids the homeless to
enter the kitchen is saying, "You are dirty. I am clean. Stay away!"

In the face of such circumstances, the marginalized person
meets disharmony eye-to-eye. Already weathering or perhaps
overcome by a myriad of internal and external vulnerabilities, the
person can be pushed further to the outer fringes of disconnectedness. Our disharmony can only give birth to further apartness.

Caregiver harmony and humanistic values toward the other
is vital and necessitates ongoing critical questioning and reflection.
Most caregivers are value-centered, but need to uncover and put
their beliefs into practice so they can express giving, nurturing,

and valuing. Our intention needs to drive us to unite ourselves with the person in spite of severe behavioral problems. We need to communicate peace to the person, even in the most disruptive of times. While we prevent harm, we need to find words, gestures, and other forms of contact that signal ourselves as safe harbors, not the confusion of storms. We need to use our hands, eyes, and words to give value in spite of the other's disharmony. This is not an easy process. Although most would agree with these concepts, it is hard to be consistent with them when being hit, spat upon, kicked, or cursed. Our values can easily fly out the window when confronted with such acts. Obviously, it is quite difficult to maintain, let alone deepen our values, when under attack. However, it is during these moments that the process calls on us to be at our best.

Ebb and Flow

Passing through these worst moments, we move into a dimension in which the other conveys some degree of harmony. It appears and then disappears like the ebb and flow of the sea, with harmony driven ever more forcefully by the undercurrent of unconditional valuing. The person is battling against years of distrust. For an instant, trust shows itself and then fades. These appearances become longer, and the distrust, weaker. As we see slight changes, we might think that all is well. Yet the growth process goes in spurts; moving closer is followed by some distancing.

It is especially important to signal valuing at difficult moments, but it is necessary that it always be present and seen as a life pattern. We are initiators of new meanings, which at the start make little or no sense to the other. It is crucial that we base our interactions on serenity and the knowledge that there will be an increasing coming together. Any sign of anger or oppression will quickly tell the person to rebel or withdraw more. Our perseverance results in a gradual calming and mutual harmony, but it is common for the person to swing between trust and distrust, feeling valued and then devalued. Old meanings die hard; they are entrenched. Our continuing role centers on unconditional valuing, its increasing elicitation, and the facilitation of engagement.

Bonding and Companionship

In time, the feeling of mutuality grows and deepens. The worst moments become less frequent and less intense. Dialogue is no longer so one-sided and structured; it slowly becomes more natural. We begin to see the person linger with us, become more engaged, and convey a strong possibility of mutuality. Instead of running away, the person comes toward us. Instead of tantruming, the person seeks out doing things with us. Most significantly, our words and touch are not only given, but are returned. Of course, the person is still vulnerable and will have difficult moments. But the emerging bond of friendship will diminish these times, their intensity, and their impact. We begin to feel at ease and comfortable in our knowledge that feelings of companionship are taking hold.

Interdependence

From the start, we need to include as many caregivers and others as possible in this process. One thread can make a delicate lace, yet the more threads that are intertwined, the more enduring the fabric of companionship will be. As these feelings emerge in our relationship, we need to ensure that the person also learns to reach out toward others, participate with them, and value them. Essentially, a circle of friends begins to surround the person, making each emotionally stronger and enabling each to tolerate the vicissitudes of life. This circle needs to be woven where the person lives, works, or goes to school. It is seen in small groups living together, knowing one another, and sharing their daily lives. It is seen in workplaces where men and women come together to express their talents in labor and form new friendships. It is seen in schools where children are learning to live together. Of course, beyond this circle, many will remain as strangers. Some will continue to be prejudiced, intolerant, and impatient. However, when the circle of friends is strong and stable, the vulnerable person will be able to better confront such persons. The knowledge, experience, and feeling of a network of friends helps to solidify emotional well-being. When change occurs or problems arise, this interdependence helps to recenter the person.

Luke had a history of severe aggression. He was diagnosed as having autism; hence he could not talk much and lacked many self-care skills. He would hit people with his fists, pull out their hair, and bite people. A big adolescent, he frightened most people. His caregivers' response was to physically subdue him whenever he was "noncompliant" and spray "water mist" in his face as punishment. He would become more violent during this procedure; nevertheless, they continued to do it because they felt they were in control.

Yet, looking at his life situation and the way people interacted with him, his escalating violence made sense. He was drowning in the midst of an absurd and anguish-filled world. His disharmony was worsened by those around him. He lived among other marginalized people in a public institution. Caregivers had no time to be bothered by his inner suffering and left him squatting alone on the floor for long periods of time. He gazed at the other lost people, heard their moans, and watched the controllers carry out their programs. When his turn came to be told what to do and where to do it, he would react slowly and reluctantly and would rebel. He sensed that participation was fruitless since it would only result in cold reward. His caregivers could tell when he was about to become angry since aggression was always preceded by clear physical signs: rocking, hyperventilation, a flushed face, and angry sounds. But they felt compliance was more important, and this would make him violent.

The alternative was to engage him in a daily routine filled with valuing. He needed structure, compromise, and multiple opportunities to receive and learn to reciprocate valuing. He needed to know that he was safe and secure with his caregivers.

However, to do this, the caregivers needed to have an inner harmony. Someone in this almost empty world had to stand up and create new meanings for Luke. When his favorite caregiver reflected on preventing his outbursts, she made sure that she knew that her expectations were to prevent violence as much as possible and to engage and value him.

On the first day, she sat at a table across from him. When he tossed the material onto the floor, she ignored it and continued dialoguing. She made certain that she only used her hands to warmly help or value him so that he could begin to grasp their meaning as instruments of valuing. When he started rocking, she told him not to worry and to take a momentary break while she completed the activity.

On this same day, he broke out into a flurry of aggression during a time when she had become careless. He stood up, tossed tables and chairs, jumped up and down, and grabbed her hair. She continued to dialogue and reach up to his hand which was twined in her hair. She asked for a handshake, and he released his grasp and after a few seconds shook her hand. She then quickly increased her valuing and encouraged his participation. He then gradually calmed.

Luke became more at ease with her as each hour passed. He still had difficult moments, yet each time these were less intense and less prolonged. She could see the currents of change flowing toward companionship. She knew it would be a long and hard process, but was willing to persevere.

For the first few hours, she worked with him alone. When two other caregivers started to watch, she invited them to sit and participate. Luke feared them. But the caregiver showed them what she was doing and asked them to follow her example. She explained what she was doing and why. Slowly, they introduced themselves into the process. They went through some difficult moments since Luke had no reason to feel secure with them or become engaged. Yet, with the first caregiver's help, they continued. Thus began the formation of a circle of friends.

A few hours later, they brought two other residents into the group and went through the same process. This became their model for Luke—bringing him together with other caregivers and residents. The first caregiver assumed responsibility to deepen her feelings of oneness with Luke and to help others persevere in the process. She knew that she had to focus on helping others become harmonious and to warmly help Luke. His violence diminished as their violence turned to valuing. His ability and desire to be with a growing circle of others expanded as they taught him to accept and return valuing.

Preventing Disharmony

To facilitate movement through these difficult moments, we need to focus on preventing problems before they arise. Our attention needs to be preventive in the way we approach the individual, how we express valuing, the tone of our interactions, giving value to the person many times more than we imagine necessary, and, at the same time, totally decreasing our dominative interactions. For Luke and his caregivers, this was difficult since they were so accustomed to a different relationship. Their interactions, like ours, were cold and demanding, their attention was based on compliance, and their words were spoken as if they were reading from a script. Prevention takes a different approach: greeting the person, conversing as a friend, and, if there is a task to be done, accomplishing it with the person. Or, if the person is in the midst of a fury, instead of seeking control, preventing further escalation calls for decreasing demands and increasing valuing.

As soon as we notice any slight indication of frustration, we have to focus more on warmly helping, ensuring a smooth flow to our interactions, and deepening the tone of our dialogue. We

---

Prevention of Disharmony
- Watch for any slight indicators
- Decrease demands
- Increase valuing
- Help the person more
- Avoid any focus on compliance
- Be nurturing
- Avoid grabbing or reprimanding
- Facilitate a smooth flow of engagement

need to battle against the compulsion for the other's obedience or finishing a task and, instead, concentrate on what we are signalling. Frequently, we need to back off and take a break with the person. Nothing is worth risking violence. As behavioral difficulties arise, we need to put in check any "natural" reactions that aggression, self-injury, or withdrawal might engender. We have to learn to tolerate alienating interactions and not permit them to make us disharmonious—angry, frustrated, or impatient. A major challenge is to avoid the escalation of violence. Decreasing demands tells the person that the reason for being together is not obedience, but to value one another. At these moments, it is paradoxical that we need to become more nurturing and give more help.

OLD MEANINGS—NEW MEANINGS

In this mutual change process, our initial task revolves around transforming what we signify to the person. When we approach the other person, what does our movement represent? What do our words convey? What does the person see in us? As we raise our hands, what does this mean to the person? The people whom we want to help possess a life history. Part of this history involves his or her vulnerability and talents, and part involves the cumulative effect of his or her past relationships. We also bring our history—our values, training, talents, and needs. The fact that we desire to bring about a different kind of relationship is generally not strong enough to cut through the layers of history. We cannot assume that our presence will represent anything different than what history has taught the person, nor can we be certain that our intention will endure violent or frustrating onslaughts unless we resolve to always question ourselves and seek support from others. In spite of our good intentions, some violence or withdrawal is almost inevitable at the start.

The formation of interdependence calls for a twofold process on our part. First, we need to dissociate all interactions and in-

Our initial responsibility in the change process is
  • To take away old meanings in ourselves and the other
  • To tolerate the alienating interactions of the other
  • To establish new meanings in ourselves and the other

dicators of emotional apartness from their previous meanings. Instead of paying attention to or feeding into acts of aggression, self-injury, or withdrawal, we need to give them no significance. This taking old meanings needs be done in a kind way that is simultaneously linked with giving new meanings. It is not what behaviorists would call "ignoring" or "extinction" because it is accompanied by the enablement of engagement and uncondi- tional valuing. Second, if the person refuses to participate, we do the activity and patiently try to engage the individual. Regardless of participation, we continue to give valuing. In essence, we are giving a different significance to our interactions filled with val- uing, safety and security, and engagement. While preventing as much violence as possible, and almost all of it is preventable, we have to be empathic and patient so that the process can take hold. Any intolerance will inevitably lead to mutual violence. We need to approach, become engaged with, and unconditionally value the person while also weathering any furies without giving them their old meanings. In this process, we have to be sensitive to the most insignificant interactions. It is insufficient to say we are going to "redirect" the person when acting out. This often equates with force, excessive demands, and the deepening of fear. Giving new meaning to and restructuring interactions necessitates mutual change. But the process has to begin with us—what we signify and how we express and enable new meanings to our presence and engagement with us. The core of this resignification is the driving power of our valuing.

Taking Away Old Meanings

When mild or major problems arise, we need to try to void them of their old symbolism. We are asked to designify the meaning of everything that historically brought about distancing. Behavior problems communicate feelings such as "I scream. You back off"; "I hit. You stop pushing"; "I swear. You send me away." We need to respect these communications, but also initiate a concurrent process that takes these old meanings away and replaces them with new ones. In essence, we recognize that the person and ourselves are symbolic of old meanings. Our presence can signal fear; our hands and words can signal demand; our movements can equate with an attack. The person interprets our presence according to past experiences. And we see the individual from their history and ours. We, too, can be filled with fear, anger, or repugnancy. Our commitment needs to lead us to eliminate these old meanings so that new symbols might begin to emerge. This includes our reactions to aggression, self-injury, or withdrawal. It also involves breaking away from objectives such as compliance. We are no longer saying, "Do this or else!" but, rather, "We will do this together because that is how I can show friendship." We are designifying the person's disruptive or destructive interactions as well as what we have historically meant. It does not mean disregarding the person; it involves creating interactions that have a totally new meaning. It partially means ignoring the particular behavior, but it is much more since it requires us to enter into the person's often hostile and rejecting space as we express valuing and effectuate engagement. But we need to honor, respect, and understand what the person is feeling within their expression of violence. At the same time, we need to communicate the feeling that a new day is at hand. We acknowledge vulnerability and history while also giving hope. We are like aliens entering a strange land in which the inhabitants have no reason to accept us and every reason to distrust us.

Teaching New Meanings

We assume a commitment to designify the disharmonious interactions that equate with apartness, while always protecting self and others; but, at the same time, our primary challenge is to

dedicate ourselves to establishing new meanings in the relationship. Our hands are no longer instruments of oppression and our
words are no longer sounds of submission. Rather, they become
signs and symbols of valuing and engagement. In many situations,
we will be rejected and at times even attacked. This understanding
includes a deepening commitment to dialogue, thereby teaching
the goodness inherent in engagement and valuing. This process is
our primary and ongoing responsibility. Giving new meanings can
be initially confusing to the person and difficult for the caregiver.
The key factor is to signal safety and security and center our
interactions on valuing.

The very state of marginalization means that the other is
unable to reach out, unwilling to be with us, and unresponsive to
any form of valuing. We are called on to represent new meanings
that involve significant change in ourselves. They are complex and
require practice and ongoing questioning. They involve an inner
struggle since we will often feel frustrated, insulted, and saddened
by the other's onslaughts. In spite of this, we are called on to
increasingly express value toward the person. In the first dimensions of this process, we need to be acutely aware of the series of
choices that are before us.

Caregiver Choices in the First Dimensions of Change	
Old Meanings	*New Meanings*
Disharmony	Harmony
Cold Assistance	Warm Assistance
Restraint	Warm Protection
Contingent Reward	Unconditional Valuing
Unilateral Reward-Giving	Elicitation of Valuing
Clientship	Companionship
Self-Reliance	Mutual Participation
Rigidity	Flexibility
Phoniness	Authenticity
Monologue	Dialogue
Aloofness	Spiritedness
Independence	Interdependence

When the person is enraged, or simply apart from us, we need to represent harmony, avoiding any domineering interactions and conveying unconditional acceptance. At these moments, if we cannot express serenity, then we need not expect it in the other. The person's emotional well-being is in our hands. If we want to enable any form of engagement, the expression of our warmth will help tell the person that our hands and words are different. If aggression or self-injury are the person's answer to our proximity, we still need to symbolize a feeling of nonviolence. And any feeling of "I will only reward you if you are behaving well!" will invariably conjure up the ghosts of the past. Our being with the other needs to give clear and strong messages that this is a mutual process in which we are both becoming more. We need to make sure that we are perceived as equals with the person instead of signalling a message of authority or independence. We cannot follow lock-step prescriptions or behavioral contracts for authenticity will become lost. Our central role is to express unconditional valuing through dialogue and extend this spirit toward as many others as possible. At every moment, we need to be weighing the degree and intensity of what we represent to the person. We have to be the enduring ones. The resignification process means that we enter a process of change before expecting any change in the other. It is often a slow and difficult process and one in which we need to measure our movement toward other-centeredness in a number of different variables.

New meanings versus old meanings. When we look toward new meanings, our actions are focused on creating, enabling, and bringing about interdependent modes of interactions with no focus on distancing interactions other than those that protect the person or others from harm. All our interactions begin with, center on, and lead to human valuing. When we look to old meanings, our intentions and actions are geared to the distancing interactions and controlling or managing "maladaptive" behaviors.

Harmony versus disharmony. When we're in harmony we are warmer, more valuing, and protective without restraining, especially when acts of aggression, self-injury, or withdrawal arise. When we're in disharmony we are nervous, frustrated, and angered when such acts occur, and we resort to forms of restraint or contingency, or just give up.

Warm help versus restraint. When we are warm our interactions transmit a feeling of authenticity whenever we are trying to help the person participate. We show warmth in the way we physically help, with the tone of our words, and our nonverbal communication. When we are cold our interactions are mechanistic or bossy, for example, in ordering the person to do something, grabbing their hands to make them do it, or giving looks that seem distancing.

Warm protection versus cold protection. In warm protection, we protect the person or others from harm in a manner that does not use force, does not immobilize, and does not make the person more fearful or angrier. Examples of warm protection are blocking hits with our forearm instead of grabbing or yelling and shadowing self-hits with our arm or hand. In cold protection our interactions lead to anger and fear, and seem as though we are bent on ordering the person around or desiring sheer obedience. Examples of cold protection are actions such as grabbing a person's fist, yelling at the person, or restraining the person through physical or environmental arrangements.

Unconditional valuing versus contingent reward. When we value someone unconditionally, our words, gestures, and physical interactions express friendship, sharing, and interdependence in an ongoing manner regardless of how the person is interacting or what he or she is doing. Unconditional valuing fully occurs when we continue to express praise, honor, and respect during good moments and bad. During the worst times, it often is expressed through nurturing interactions such as saying warmly, "That's fine. I know you don't feel good. You just rest a minute and I'll help!" When we use contingent reward we primarily give praise or material rewards for good deeds done; we wait until the person earns our praise or attention. Unless the person does something that we want, we do not communicate valuing at all.

Elicitation of valuing versus one-sided value-giving. When we elicit value while we give unconditional valuing, we are trying to get the person to respond with valuing toward ourselves through their words, gestures, or physical interactions. If the person is nonverbal, we try to help the person to smile, reach out, and communicate feelings of union. If the person is verbal, we key in on conversation that signals a common ground and elicit verbal and nonverbal expressions of union. When value-giving is one-sided, we perhaps give a lot of unconditional reward, but we do not seek or expect valuing from the person. We are the giver, and the marginalized person is the receiver.

Companionship versus clientship. With companionship we regard the person as our friend and as an equal who is filled with gifts and talents. We approach the person as our brother or sister, seeing no distinction in value or worth due to his or her diagnosis, behaviors, or history. Indeed, we recognize that their very mar-ginalization beckons us to reach out as a companion. With client-ship we view the person as someone to be "treated," "modified," or "programmed." We see the person as a problem, a diagnosis, or a behavioral situation. Examples include calling the person a "run-ner" or a "spitter." Also included are gestures, facial expressions, and tones of voice that are cold, condescending, or authoritarian, and actions such as supervising meals instead of eating with the person or having a staff party and a client party.

Mutual participation versus self-reliance. When we engage in mutual participation we do activities, tasks, and daily events with the person. Although we also seek to teach new skills so that the person might develop his or her talents to the fullest, our primary focus is not on skill acquisition or correctness, but on being together and doing things with the person. When we en-courage self-reliance our central posture is one of getting the person to do things for the sake of doing them, to do things correctly, and to become independent. Self-reliance involves telling the person to get something done while we stand or sit and watch and wait.

Flexibility versus rigidity. When we are flexible we accept the ebb and flow of interests, give choices, and respect and honor the verbal and nonverbal messages that the person expresses. We are willing to back off and are sensitive to precursors to nervousness, anger, or fear. Flexibility is seen when we give the person a few moments to rest, give more help, or just say, "The heck with it! Let's do something else!" When we are rigid we feel the person has to do what we want him or her to do, when we want and in the manner we want. We do not back off and are not sensitive to precursors to behavioral upheavals, and push on regardless.

Authenticity versus phoniness. Authentic interactions are filled with genuine positive regard for the person, expressing warmth naturally and spontaneously. We feel at ease in our helping and dialogue. We express ourself, our feelings, our thoughts, our emotions, and our interests to the person. Phony interactions are a role being played and follow a programmed plan. Our physical movements, our words, and our gestures are robot-like.

Dialogue versus monologue. When we dialogue we are expressing our own thoughts and feelings: telling stories and conversing about friendship and interdependence: and evoking similar thoughts and feelings from the person, in a genuine, ongoing flow, regardless of what the person is doing. It is the deepest way to express unconditional valuing. When we monologue we are carrying on a conversation that is neither personalized to our own reality nor to the person's. Monologue often relates to just the task being done, compliance, or deeds accomplished.

Spiritedness versus aloofness. When we are spirited we evoke a feeling of playfulness, joy, and empathy in our interactions. Even when sharing serious themes, we place ourselves in the same reality as the person: when the person suffers, we share our suffering; when the person rejoices, we share our joys. When we are aloof we carry out interventions and follow schedules. Only orderliness and efficiency, not the person, seems to matter. When we're aloof, we show a spirit of drabness or apartness.

Expanded relationships versus dependence. In expanded relationships, we create a feeling of connectedness beyond ourselves and the person, and the person feels safe and secure with or without our immediate presence because others have entered the process. We draw them into our relationship and help the person reach out to them. With dependence we create an overprotective relationship with the person and do not extend the relationship beyond ourselves, and the person only interacts well if we are physically present.

These are the various elements which we need to reflect on during the initial disharmony and its subsequent reappearances as the process ebbs and flows. Our task is to evoke the new meanings that signal oneness and rupture apartness. A marked tendency toward domination will exist, pushing and pulling us into an attitude of control. Our struggle is to initiate the resignification process by first looking at ourselves. There will be no new meanings until we change. It is most helpful to work with others, critique our interactions, and increasingly put our values into practice. Our responsibility is multifaceted and requires ongoing personal changes and a quest to represent value-centered interactions.

CONCLUSION

Caregiving is a life project that involves more than helping others. It means transforming ourselves, what we represent, and how we express these new meanings to marginalized people. It also involves a growing understanding of the causes of marginalization, the subtle and gross signals that our interactions and our institutions can convey, and the social change that needs to occur. Reflecting on ourselves, we need to make sure that every move we make represents new meanings. This requires us to spend time with the other and be tolerant of disharmony. As we undergo change, we simultaneously help the other to accompany us. What had been violence becomes harmony. What had been apartness and alienation becomes companionship and interdependence. At the same time, we need to begin to look at the world around us—family, school, group home, ward, workplace, shelter—and discover ways to draw others into the change process.

Chapter 8
THE PRACTICE OF
MUTUAL CHANGE

Several supportive techniques can be mobilized to effectuate and intensify the mutual change process. In assuming responsibility for this change, caregivers need to have the skills to enable the establishment of feelings of companionship. This is much easier said than done since each marginalized individual brings unique emotional challenges to the situation. Some might fear the caregiver and rebel against any interactions. Others might be consumed by an overwhelming sadness and withdraw from any contact. Some individuals will be mentally ill, others, mentally retarded, and still others, aged. Some will have strong supportive networks while others will be alone and abandoned. Some will be destitute, unemployed, and homeless while others will have material goods and yet still be burdened by feelings of apartness.

Unlike many current practices, these techniques are applied in various combinations at different instances. There is no cookbook formula that indicates, "Do this, then do that . . ." There is no easy method as to how to bring about feelings of companionship. The change process involves arduous work, flexibility, and creativity. The driving force always needs to be unconditional valuing, but to convey this requires an array of techniques. Caregivers should be careful to avoid simple solutions. These techniques call for hard work, decision making from one moment to the next, and the willingness to persevere. Caregivers need to constantly question their values and search for the right combination of techniques to bring about feelings of security, engagement, and valuing.

We need to be ready to prevent violence whenever possible and deal with it nonviolently when it arises. Some of the techniques help to prevent or diminish violence. Others help to increase participation. And still others help to center our interactions on valuing. They comprise a dynamic, ever-changing approach.

SUPPORTIVE TECHNIQUES

Most of the supportive techniques are common psychological and educational practices, and their worth lies in their use as ways to enable and support valuing interactions through mutual engagement while also preventing violence. Their basic purpose is to give caregivers the opportunity to express feelings of security, to teach the importance of mutual engagement, and to deepen the meaning of being valued and valuing others.

Errorless teaching enables us to bring about mutual participation. Initially, it is often helpful for caregivers to structure their interactions with the individual through the use of tasks and activities. These bring us into direct contact with the person and help link our value-giving to engagement with us. Whatever the activity might be, we need to facilitate participation and give whatever help the person might need. To make certain that the person does not become frustrated, tasks should be made as easy as possible. As the person becomes more engaged, then we can make the activities more complex and more skill-oriented. Any way we can avoid confusion or frustration helps maintain the focus on mutual participation. To enable this involves split-second decisions and changes. In the beginning, the slightest error can be frustrating and lead to violence. We have to be ever-ready to ensure that the interactions flow smoothly.

Task analysis supports errorless teaching. It involves breaking down tasks and activities so that we can proceed more easily

---

Supportive Techniques

- Errorless teaching: to facilitate participation, decrease frustration, and highlight value-giving.
- Task analysis: to facilitate participation through simplification and decrease difficulties in participation.
- Environmental arrangements: to prevent behavioral difficulties and increase participation.
- Warm helping: to express valuing in the process of enabling participation.
- Co-participation with the person: to symbolize and practice equality by being with and working with the person, to facilitate participation, and to increase feelings of engagement.
- Use of tasks and activities as vehicles for engagement: to keep the focus on the relationship.
- Identification of behavioral precursors: to prevent behavioral difficulties before they become serious or decrease their intensity or duration.
- Reduction of verbal and physical instructions: to increase the focus on valuing and dialogue and decrease domination.
- Choice-making: to increase the person's feeling of freedom and decrease frustration.
- Fading direct help: to increase individual talents by enabling the person to self-initiate and maintain participation and engagement.
- Dialogue: to increase feelings of interdependence, unconditional valuing, and its reciprocation.

---

and do not have to be concerned with what comes next. Thus it facilitates participation. The more we can enable a smooth flow when doing activities with the marginalized person, the more likely he or she will participate with us. By breaking down one task into small, easily attainable tasks, we become more flexible and signal that task completion is not the primary goal but rather mutual participation. For example, if we see that the person is becoming frustrated or nervous, we can simplify the task, give more warm help, and let the person know that mutually valuing interactions are more important than the particular task. Or if we feel that the person is participating well, we can make the task more complicated while at the same time increasing our dialogue and the elicitation of valuing.

Making sure that the environment is conducive to participation and the prevention of aggression and self-injury is important. This technique includes such considerations as where we sit or stand, how we approach the person, how we offer warm help, how we enable participation, and how we give and elicit valuing. These arrangements can change from one second to the next. At one moment it might be necessary to sit at a table across from an aggressive person. But as calming and participation occur, we might quietly move closer. Or if someone is accustomed to banging his or her head on tables, we might start without a table and then gradually introduce one to the person. Environmental arrangements should not be permanent or involve placing individuals apart from others. The environment should facilitate valuing interactions between the caregiver and the individual and should never promote any feelings of restraint or domination. Environmental arrangements can involve complex changes such as taking a person out of a dehumanizing setting and placing him or her in a family-like environment. Some institutional settings are so wretched that they prevent supportive techniques from being helpful.

In warmly helping the individual, we concentrate on making our words and touch as supportive, nondemanding, and valuing as possible. Since the person is likely fearful, we need to express warmth especially in those interactions that have been historically equated with demands. Indeed, our helping needs to signal the feeling that we are friends. For example, if we are handing an item to someone, every movement of ours needs to convey a spirit of mutuality. We also need to avoid expressing insistence or demands. The idea is not to make the person do something, but to enable mutual engagement. One way to facilitate engagement is to interlace our helping with valuing. For example, if a caregiver would like an individual to help wash the dishes, and the person refuses, the caregiver might start washing them alone but while initiating a conversation with the person. As the person becomes attentive, the caregiver might try to encourage the person to put away the dried dishes. Warm helping involves an ongoing focus on mutual engagement, not skill acquisition or task completion. It avoids any focus on compliance or obedience. How we help is a reflection of ourselves and affects how the person interprets our relationship with him or her and our purpose.

The soundest way to warmly help someone is through co-participation. Instead of standing over someone like as straw boss with our arms folded, we need convey that we will accomplish the activity with the marginalized person. Since our primary purpose is to teach human engagement and valuing, the task at hand is simply a vehicle for enabling participation and a means to structure our valuing. Co-participation not only decreases the likelihood of frustrations arising out of mistakes or difficulty in doing the activity, but it conveys a strong message of solidarity. As we participate side by side with the person, we can carry out a dialogue. In this, we need to avoid any expression of authoritarian feelings and give instructions in a "we" form. For example, if we want an aggressive child to do a school task, we might sit next to him or her, initiate a conversation, and begin doing the particular task without making any demands. As the child calms, we could then weave a comment into the dialogue such as, "It is good to work together. Doing things together means we are becoming friends." If he or she is nervous or does not wish to participate, we need to heighten our participation and clearly convey the feeling that it is good to be with the child. Engagement with us is the purpose. The only way to teach the goodness of doing projects together is to do them with the person.

Tasks and activities provide a structure for caregivers in their attempt to bring about engagement. When someone is aggressive, self-injurious, or withdrawn, we need a way to create a common ground between ourselves and the marginalized person. Tasks and activities can serve as a bridge to this common ground. They can help us focus on the emerging relationship since we can use them to bring us together with the person, demonstrate our solidarity, and create dialogue. It is important to put aside any primary focus on skill acquisition. Tasks are often used to teach new skills, but this is of secondary importance. Although at first the individual sees little or no meaning in human engagement, tasks will teach him or her the meaning of participation.

Aggression and self-injury are almost always preceded by warning signs. Individuals often begin to appear confused, frustrated, or disoriented. They show signs of nervousness, frustration, or anger. Their speech might become more rapid or garbled. Their faces might become tense and flushed. Their hands might begin to tremble. We need to become sensitive to these precursors to violence and avoid pushing the individual into deeper anguish. Caregivers often feel compelled to increase demands and decrease their unconditional valuing during the worst moments. However, upon seeing these signs, it is helpful to back off from any demands, give more warm help, increase valuing, and convey feelings of patience and tolerance.

Interactions between caregivers and marginalized individuals frequently consist of instructions like "Do this, then do that!" We often order people around as if they have no value, no feelings, and no equality with us. Instructions often equate with demands. An authoritarian relationship almost always elicits violence. The creation of feelings of engagement requires the expression of an equal relationship, one of sisterhood or brotherhood. Any instructions need to be woven into our dialogue with the individual and convey a sense of mutuality. If the individual needs physical help to participate, this should also be done in a warm and non-demanding manner. If we take a person by the hand to help do a particular activity, our hand should convey valuing and warmth. The slightest indication of demand can send a strong signal to the person that we are interested in obedience instead of a mutually valuing relationship.

From the start, it is helpful to present choices to the person in order to give a sense of mutuality. However, we also need to remember that the individual often will have no desire to do anything with us. Choice making grows as the individual begins to feel more secure with us. When there is little or no participation, the choices we present need always lead to participation with us. Our role is to facilitate participation even in the face of rejection. If we approach an individual and ask, "Do you want to help me clean the floor," and the person runs away or refuses, then we have painted ourselves into a corner. We need to remember that engagement with us is more critical than choice making. Thus, instead of asking whether someone wants to help clean the floor, we might ask, "Which can we do together, clean the floor or wash the windows?" Here are two choices and our role is to facilitate one in spite of any refusal. This does not mean insisting that one be done. It means that we have to increase our warm helping, value giving, and co-participation in order to bring about one of the options. As the person learns that it is good to participate with us, choice making will become more meaningful.

As time passes and participation becomes easier, we need to "fade" our presence so as not to make the person overly dependent on us. A helpful strategy is to momentarily leave the person and then return while he or she is still doing the activity instead of leaving upon completion or when stopping. The basic teaching purpose is to engage the person, not complete a task. Sometimes fading is much more subtle. It might involve giving less help or increasing our expectations of how much the person can participate.

And, as we have said repeatedly, unconditional valuing in the form of dialogue needs to be at the center of our interactions with the marginalized person. Our dialogue with the person is the driving force of what we do and what we represent. It involves our conversation, movements, gestures, and physical contact with the person. We frequently stop giving value when the individual becomes belligerent or nonparticipatory. Yet we need to increase our dialogue at the worst moments. This ongoing valuing does not mean constant chatter. It does mean a continuous expression of warm and genuine solidarity.

The choice of these techniques at any particular moment

depends upon answering the question, "Which techniques will increase valuing and decrease domination?" The establishment of companionship and feelings of interdependence is a flexible process and requires decision-making in the very act of caregiving— not at a distant meeting. What we express, what we do, and how we react depends upon the moment.

> Jim slides onto the floor when he sees his teacher approach. The teacher sits on the floor next to him and speaks to him as a friend. Jim tries to throw spelling practice sheets to the floor. She scoots them aside. Jim responds by swinging his fist, and she receives the blow on her arm. Then Jim crawls under the table. She moves with him and stays at Jim's side to avoid being forcefully hit. But the entire time she is facilitating participation on the particular task just by placing a practice sheet in Jim's hand and accepting it back from him. Plus she continues to dialogue throughout this process. She has to hold onto each sheet with her fingers and, at the same time, avoids grabbing. Her movements are in unison with Jim's as the child tries to fling the paper. Then she spells out a particular word for Jim. A few minutes later Jim is sitting up. He is on the floor, but participating more and giving her handshakes. She starts to give less help and elicit more valuing. A moment later Jim screams and kicks. She gives more help and more soothing valuing. As Jim calms, the teacher sits on a nearby chair and Jim sits beside her.

It the caregiver had to follow a rigid plan, it is likely that Jim would not have started to participate, nor would the caregiver have been able to center her interactions on valuing. In this brief time, the teacher made multiple decisions, all based on engagement and valuing. So at any particular moment we have to be ready to vary these supportive techniques, always keeping in mind that our commitment has to revolve around decreasing any domineering interactions and dramatically increasing our value-giving. These are often subtle interactions such as smiling instead of frowning, doing activities with the person instead of ordering them done, going to wherever the person might be instead of escorting the individual to where we want her or him to be, being concerned with enabling participation and dialogue instead of worrying about being manipulated or reinforcing inappropriate behaviors, and warmly gazing instead of looking through the person. These techniques gradually help to bring about the understandings and feelings that our presence represents: safety, mutual participation, and valuing.

ENGAGEMENT AS A MEANS FOR VALUING AND SHARING

As we center our interactions on valuing and resignifying the relationship using a variety of these supportive techniques, many challenges can arise at any particular moment. Since the person will often reject us, if not fear us, and since our valuing will hold little, if any, meaning, we need to generate ways to effectuate engagement, an emotional coming toward us even while the person is turning away or fighting. Being with someone is much more than physical proximity. It involves finding ways to bring about participation, express valuing, and teach others to share.

Facilitating Participation

As we try to bring about participation, we have to make sure that our every movement reflects warmth: approach serenely, be

---

To facilitate participation and prevent interactional difficulties
- Reflect on how you can express warmth from the first moment
- Find activities that are of long duration, fit the age of the person, are useful in daily life, and encourage coming together
- Regard these activities primarily as a way to structure interactions
- Arrange the setting and activities
- Think about where the setting would be best in relation to the person

prepared to stay with the person, and be ready to move to wherever the person might go. It is helpful to have activities that will last a long period since the more the person is with us, the more we will be able to give value. A momentary lapse can break the flow of participation. The focus needs to be on being engaged with us, not the task. At every moment, we also need to be considering what might prevent violence. This requires foresight, preparation, and endurance on our part.

A Flow of Participation

Since we are often confronted with frequent periods of withdrawal or disruption, we need to ensure a smooth flow of participation. The smoother participation is, the less likely the person will become upset. This calls for our direct and ongoing involvement in the activity and our smoothing out rough moments. Each second is critical since a moment of distraction can lead to upheaval. What facilitates at one point might not at another so flexibility is necessary. It is also helpful to avoid a fixation on the task or the person's ability to accomplish it. The focus needs to be on participating with us. The fact that the person might know how to do something is irrelevant. If the activity is not being done, our responsibility is to facilitate and enable engagement with us. We often presume too much in relation to emotional stability when we arrogantly pronounce, "He just does not want to do it!" We might think that because a person can do something, we ought to be able to lessen our help. However, in the beginning, it is better to provide too much help rather than too little.

We also need to be alert to the ebb and flow of disharmony. At any sign of turmoil, our role involves simplifying what is being done or doing it ourselves to maintain the flow. We become modulators whenever the smallest indicators of nervousness or sadness occur. For example, if the person starts to scream and hyperventilate, we need to slow our words and movements, thereby helping the person to moderate his or her feelings. Although choice might not make such sense, since the individual has little or no desire to interact with us, it is good to always present options.

To facilitate a flow of participation
- Simplify the particular task so that the entire focus is on participation
- As participation flows, then consider more complex activities
- If turmoil is about to occur, slow down, simplify activities further, or back off for a moment
- No matter what happens, keep your focus on valuing and mutual engagement
- Have at least 2–3 activities available at any moment, but avoid overwhelming the person
- If the person slows down, animate him or her; if he or she becomes overly excited, slow down
- Avoid grabbing the person, even in a slight way, in order to enable participation
- Avoid giving just verbal instructions to enable participation; if you have to give them, do so within the dialogue
- If participation is nonexistent, help the person by increasing your valuing, making it more sincere and warm, and do the activity with the person—even if you are doing almost all of it

If the person refuses to do anything, we need to continue to center most of our interactions on bringing about participation.

Diminishing Violence

Should the flow of participation be disrupted, we then have to deal with the likelihood of the person becoming aggressive or self-injurious. We need to see this emerging and find ways to prevent further escalation so that intense valuing can stay at the center of our interactions. We have to sense when the person is becoming disengaged. Clear indications of this are more rapid speech, rocking, trembling, looking about anxiously, moaning, and lessening the level of participation. If any of these occur, we need to slow down and increase warmly helping. The need for our help varies—sometimes more, sometimes less—and depends on the mood of the moment. We need to maintain a steady level of engagement with us. When nervousness occurs, slowing down the

To diminish the probability of the escalation of aggression or self-injury
- Slow down the particular activity, but try not to stop
- Keep the focus on giving and eliciting value
- Stay warm, tolerant, forebearing, and affectionate
- If the person flails his arms, back off momentarily, but continue to express valuing
- If the person is about to hit you or self, simply shadow or block the hit with your hand or arm. Avoid grabbing or ordering the person to stop
- If the person is moving around, stay a step ahead and keep enabling participation and giving valuing

flow of participation can help the person calm down. Our movements and words can help modulate and decrease a worsening mood. Contrary to what often happens, we should give more help and valuing at these difficult moments. This centers the participation on the relationship instead of the activity. Sometimes, it is beneficial to simply back off and say, "You know we do not have to do this. Let's take a break!" And, at these moments, we have to continue to express valuing. If violence occurs, we should say nothing about it and continue to direct our interactions toward engagement and valuing. If we are attentive, we can foresee the potential emergence of anger and subsequently decrease our demands, increase our help, and intensify our dialogue.

Expressing Warmth and Valuing

Clearly, during these potentially disharmonious moments, we need to root our actions firmly in valuing. Yet this is most difficult to do. It requires us to question our practices in relation to our values, always making sure that our beliefs are consistent with our actions. Our intensity of interacting goes far beyond what we would normally expect. Our perception of who the person is and our purpose for engaging ourselves with the individual is vital. The driving force needs to be valuing and to increasingly link this with engagement. We need to bear in mind that our words and other ways of interacting should be centered on the person. We are saying, "You are somebody!" in spite of what might be transpiring. And we have to avoid any tendency to only value and acknowledge the person's worth for deeds done.

Since the emergence of dialogue is a complex process, we need to be sensitive to the slightest expression of our feelings reflected in changes in affect, tone of voice, and body movement. Throughout this process, we have to fight against any frustration and focus on conveying authentic and genuine positive regard. We are asked to tolerate much and give much. Our dialogue should come out of our interests and our understanding of the person's reality. Although it is difficult in the beginning, it is helpful to reflect on what animates us. If we share our own life interests with the other, we are ensured of warm and authentic expressions.

We should not be concerned with nonparticipation; rather, our focus is to bring about simply being with us. For example, if a

---

To express warm, affectionate, and personal valuing
- Value the wholeness of the person, not the task or work
- Avoid giving value only after the person has "accomplished" something
- In order to facilitate dialogue, "read" the person, closely observing subtle interactions that reflect interest, reciprocation, or a spirit of wanting to share
- Be authentic and genuine
- Increase your valuing many times over what you might think is necessary
- Search out and create distinct forms of dialogue such as story telling, jokes, reflective conversations about feelings and the human condition, and singing
- For those who have trouble participating, especially focus on giving value for any movement toward minimal participation— even if you have to do almost all of the activity for or with the person

profoundly retarded person withdraws into a fetal position, our
task is to do almost everything to find minute ways for the person
to participate. If the person has every skill imaginable but still does
not participate, our task is the same: to initially create a structure
for engagement at any level and link that structure with our valuing.

Eliciting Valuing

As difficult as it might be, we also need to continue a focus on
the elicitation of valuing. We want to equalize the relationship
through mutual valuing, no matter what might be happening.
Although difficult, we should elicit valuing during good moments
and bad. The emergence of new meaning is very much based on
the degree to which the person feels one with us. From the start,
we need to include this feeling as part of our interactions in simple
ways, such as asking for handshakes and smiles. If we convey a
strong feeling of warmth, the person will better sense our authenticity and will more likely reciprocate valuing. This does not mean
that we have to be loud or expansive; it does mean that we need
to be genuine. Our expression should be natural. Each should feel
comfortable in the way valuing is given and elicited. Also, our
interactions should be filled with surprises. There is no reason to
become smugly fixated on what the individual is supposed to do.
It is helpful to convey a sense of, "We are more important than the
activity!" Once the person feels somewhat safe with us, the elicita-

---

To elicit valuing from the person
- As you give value, seek to elicit it from the person in the form
  of handshakes, smiles, hugs, "fives," thumbs-up
- Use concrete and warm facial and corporal expressions
- Every now and then, just stop and enjoy being with the person
- If a person becomes nervous, increase value elicitation as a way
  of resignifying the interaction and calming the person
- Interpret emotional expressions or physical movements that
  might be indicative of the reciprocation of valuing

tion of valuing can also serve to interrupt violence. When a person raises a hand to slap us, we might say, "How about a handshake!" and place our hand in the individual's. This often makes sense to the person and provides a concrete alternative to violence. The elicitation of valuing requires us to interpret slight changes in the person's tone, movements, gestures, and other forms of communication so that we are alert to the slightest indication that the person might reciprocate valuing.

Expanding the Relationship

From the beginning, we need to ensure that the person expands their feelings of companionship to other persons. Friendship is not instantly transferred from one person to another, it needs to be cultivated. It is important to develop a firm emotional foundation and help create a circle of friends, since the more companions there are, the less likely emotional upheavals will occur. In addition, we need to avoid an overly dependent relationship.

The formation of a circle of friends expands outwardly—first with ourself, then two or three others, then many more. This expansion enables the person to have the feeling of a safe harbor. The individual is better able to tolerate the vicissitudes of life outside the circle. The person's life situation is bolstered by this circle of friends and the feeling of being in the community and of it rather than being a strange person in a strange land.

The start of this circle is the initial invitation of one or two others to participate along with the person. This needs to be carefully orchestrated. It can involve bringing others into physical proximity, doing an activity together, or sharing dialogue with these others.

To initiate this process, we need to first decrease the need for our actual presence. This fading process needs to start in subtle ways from the beginning, for example, being flexible and change-oriented, scooting away for a moment while participation is occurring, and increasing the person's endurance in activities. The

To extend the person beyond your relationship
- Gradually remove yourself while participation is occurring
- Increase your valuing from a distance
- Be sure to return before participation stops
- Keep your eyes open for any "slow down" and give whatever help might be necessary to keep a smooth flow going
- Share with the person what you are doing or will do
- Include the above process as part of the dialogue
- Invite 1–2 others to participate with the person and you
- Realize that this is a complex emotional process for all involved
- Beforehand, role-play how you can facilitate sharing
- Use a task as a vehicle to "work together"—one helping the other and all valuing one another
- Assume responsibility for the flow
- If one slows down, help out

more the individual participates, the easier it is to remove ourselves for a few moments and then longer.

While fading, we need to increase our verbal valuing from a distance, letting the person know that we are near and are still sources of ongoing valuing. It is helpful to return to the person several times and continue participating to let him or her know that engagement is more vital than completing an activity. When the person seems to be slowing down his activity, return and give more warm help. We should let the person know what we are doing and why, always making sure that the person feels equally valued, whether we are present or not.

As engagement occurs, we need to bring one or two others into the process. At first, it is helpful to use an activity for this coming together, but also enable each to value one another. Our task is to facilitate this complex process by working with the group, assuming responsibility for the flow of participation, and inviting each person to value the others. Our primary role is to be a model for mutual valuing. In essence, the feelings between us and the other are transformed into similar feelings among others.

Personalizing the Process

Lastly, we need to recognize that just as we have feelings, distinct personalities, and histories of life experiences, so, too, does the marginalized person. Each brings a unique life history to the interactional context. We need to empathize with this individuality, temper it when necessary, and respect the individual while enabling the mutual change process.

Many individuals will have such a strong need for affection that they become overly dependent. They might cling to us to seek too much attention. We need to deeply respect their hunger, but also make sure that we help them express it in socially acceptable ways. For example, we might want to permit exaggerated hugs for a while in a person who has been denied human contact for years or who has never learned how to express affection; but soon we should transform these into handshakes or pats on the back. Part of our responsibility is to enable individuals to survive in a community, and this involves the teaching appropriate behavior. Marginalized individuals often lack moderation in their interactions. Once feeling solidarity, they might be unable to distinguish that what is appropriate in one situation is inappropriate in another. For example, the teacher might encourage a hug from a child upon leaving school at the end of the day, but the child might do this in a grocery store with a stranger. So, the caregiver has to teach the child when and where interactions are appropriate. For those who are authoritarian, we need to consider setting limits

---

Relating with Various Personalities
- If the person is overly dependent, focus on appropriate social expressions without being offensive.
- If the person is authoritarian, focus on creating dialogue that reflects equality.
- If the person is afraid, be especially kind, warm, and nurturing.
- If the person is aggressive or self-injurious, protect yourself, the person, and others without being dominative or intolerant.

without causing a clash. Just as we do not want to lord over others, so, too, we need to help others equalize their relationship with us.

Others are fearful and cringe at our contact. We need to slowly and gently teach them to accept our touch, our words, and our gestures. Sadly, some hurt themselves or attack others. Our first task is to protect them from harm without punishment or restraint. We need to signal exceptionally strong expressions of safety, security, and unconditional valuing. No matter what history and personality the person brings, we always need to reflect kindness, warmth, and nurturing. Our role centers on helping each person learn how to relate justly with us and then others.

CONCLUSION

The problems are the most common general situations that confront us when we try to bring about engagement. Their resolution takes commitment, experience, and an ongoing checking of our values in relation to our moment-to-moment practices. We need to be empowered to decide what to do, when to do it, and how to do it based on criteria of nonviolence and unconditional valuing. Engagement is a basic dimension in the resignification process since it brings us together. Generally, it is within this structure that we can intensify our value-giving and dialogue. The initial challenge falls on us to create and maintain a flow of participation and gradually expand it outward.

Chapter 9
SUGGESTIONS FOR COMMON SITUATIONS

We have considered the supportive techniques that we can use to prevent or diminish disharmony, signal increasing safety and security, enable engagement, and, above all, convey unconditional valuing. Their use is based on moment-to-moment decision-making on our part. A critical variable is to facilitate a coming together through effectuating participation. We cannot take on new meanings if we are not in solidarity with the person. Yet, in the initial dimension of caregiving, this is quite difficult since we are confronted with the rejection of our presence and any kind of participation with us. The strategies and techniques that we described can help us move more closely to the person. However, a nearly infinite number of questions can present themselves. The more we experience various situations, the better we will be able to select techniques. Some of those that we have encountered are presented in this chapter.

COMMON SITUATIONS

Aggression

If the person tries to hit you,

- Protect yourself as unobtrusively as you can—for example, by blocking the hit with your arm.

165

- Say nothing about the hit and keep your negative feelings in check.
- Warmly help the person participate with you.
- Sometimes back off for a few seconds.
- Do the activity with or for the person.
- Continue to dialogue.
- Give strong and authentic valuing.
- Make sure the person's day is filled with valuing and sharing to prevent or decrease future problems.

We often feel compelled to punish anyone who starts to hit us. We need to ask ourselves what we represent to the person and make sure that we signal safety and security. The preponderance of aggression is predictable. The person who lashes out likely has a pattern of such behavior; plus, in any given instance, there are almost always signs that indicate violence will likely occur if interactions (or lack of interactions) continue as they are. When these predictable signs emerge, it is important to redirect the person before an act of actual aggression erupts; but, if it does, the best option is to continue to give value. We then move through these difficult moments and plan on more sensitive prevention strategies so that the aggression does not happen again or happens less intensely.

Furies

If the person is beyond participation at the moment,

- If possible, in a nurturing and calm manner, try to re-engage the person.
- If not immediately possible, protect yourself, the person, and others by making environmental arrangements, such as pushing aside tables and chairs, until the fury subsides.
- At the peak of violence, do not chastise the person; remain valuing.
- As it subsides or momentarily abates, gently re-engage the person on a task or activity and continue to dialogue.

- As the person becomes slightly involved, focus on the mutual participation so that you can maximize the feeling of union.
- Henceforth, focus on prevention by identifying the interactional and physiological signs that led up to the fury.
- As these precursors begin to appear, increase your valuing and give more warm help.

We do not have to chastise a person for an emotional fury, nor restrain them. The important thing is to help the individual know that we signal safety and security. If a person is hitting him- or herself, it is better to shadow the self-aggression by using our hands or arms to protect ourselves or others while re-engaging the person. The key is to continue the valuing and dialogue. If the person lashes out, we should calmly move out of arm's reach—for example, moving to the other side of a table or chair.

It is always necessary to remember that it is our own reactions, based on the strength of our personal posture, that will primarily increase or decrease another person's rage. This process gives us the opportunity to focus on valuing the person instead of controlling. We need to put aside any tendency to fight violence with violence. Caregivers often want to jump in with almost lethal force, and they are trained in a multitude of control procedures. We need to do away with these procedures and replace them with valuing and engagement.

Precursors to Furies

If the person is working up to a fury,

- Identify the precursors that lead up to a possible fury in order to prevent it.
- Talk to the person in a nurturing and calm manner and indicate a concrete goal, e.g., "Let's do one more. I'll even do it for you!"
- Remove unnecessary objects from around the person to avoid material being thrown or destruction of property.

- Help the person continue to participate through warm gestural or physical assistance, or even do the task for the person. Remember engagement, whether active or passive, is a major focus. Forget about compliance.
- Take a short break with the person, if helpful.
- As the signs subside, gently go back to an activity or task; this will give you some structure for increased valuing and participation.

These responses are primarily preventive. We need to strive to cut off violence before it emerges. This is vital since little good can occur in the midst of rage. Most persons with a history of violence toward others have learned through our reactions that the best way to draw others toward or away from themselves is to act out. Our punishment or restraint can easily become their reward or their way of having some power over absurd or meaningless interactions. We need to maintain the focus on teaching the person that our presence signals valuing. Unfortunately, we have a tendency to ignore precursors and push the person into a frenzy. We need to decrease demands by giving more help and increase our valuing through more sensitive dialogue.

Self-Stimulation

If the person is self-stimulating,

- If it does not interfere with human engagement, ignore it.
- If it does interfere, find a way to prevent or block it without restraining or even momentarily immobilizing the person.
- If the person is waving hands or arms, use tasks that require both hands.
- Help the person to participate by working together.
- If the person rocks, arrange the seating or table position to reduce the rocking if it is disruptive.
- Perform the task standing up, if necessary.
- Increase valuing and dialogue.

Self-stimulatory behaviors often indicate that a person is so nonparticipatory that it is more meaningful to withdraw and create one's own rewarding world. Rocking or other repetitive bodily motions bring more meaning to the person than our presence. Instead of reaching out, these individuals reach inward. There is little or no consistent positive meaning in human participation and interactions. We need to teach that human valuing is stronger and more meaningful than withdrawal. As the person learns to interact, the disruptive self-stimulating behavior will decrease. In essence, we are helping the person exchange the emptiness of self-stimulation for the fulfillment of participation.

Fear of Being with Others

If you are afraid to allow the person to go to school, work, or live with others because of the seriousness of particular behaviors,

- Teach others how to make the person feel valued.
- Teach others how to interact when and if such behaviors occur.
- Avoid placing the person near those who are defenseless, and carefully bring others into the circle.
- Develop a highly active and structured day so as to maximize opportunities for valuing and sharing.
- Teach sharing by using yourself as a model.

It is common to group people according to homogenous characteristics they share, such as grouping people with severe mental retardation together with those who have behavioral problems or persons with mild mental retardation with those exhibiting antisocial behavior. This almost inevitably creates expectations of compliance and punishment and leaves the person with few models for valuing interactions. Nations are pock-marked with camps for the alienated. Schools, group homes, and all such caregiving services need to focus on grouping together persons who are compatible with and supportive of each other.

The goal we should struggle for is that persons with special needs can associate those who are well-integrated into community life, in schools, family settings, and the like. Specifically, as we do this, we need to start to bring this person together with one or two others and orchestrate a process of sharing. One way is to use a task and have one help the other. In the beginning, we might have to sit between and facilitate every movement such as, "Now, John, hand Jim the piece. And do not forget to tell him thanks!" As we model this, each will gradually learn to share.

Refusal to Participate

If the person refuses to participate,

- Make sure there is a structured flow to the day, not just the emptiness of custodial care.
- Be aware of other caregivers who might be coaxing, cajoling, or bribing the person to participate.
- Bring about minimal participation by doing activities with the person.
- Continue to dialogue.
- Emphasize valuing and elicit it during any movement toward the slightest participation.

The major challenge in this situation is to make valuing occur, even in settings that contradict it. Many caregivers work in almost hopeless situations: institutions where the mentally retarded or mentally ill are herded like animals, nursing homes where the aged are left to fade away, homeless shelters where the poor are warehoused for an evening. Although we need to fight for social justice and establish decent places for people to live, work, and play, many caregivers still need to create hope and feelings of companionship where there is none. Thus, if we work alone in a setting that seems to be the antithesis of valuing and engagement, we have a special and difficult role: to bring hope where only despair reigns. We will often be ridiculed for our idealism and seeming naïveté. Yet we can express valuing and create feelings of companionship even in the midst of hopelessness. Our interactions are what matters. If the person in the most forsaken institutional ward runs from us and falls to the floor, we can keep on teaching the meaning of human engagement. If the person lashes out, spits, or screams at us, we can move toward him or her and continue to bring about engagement and give unconditional valuing. We are challenged to enable participation and establish feelings of solidarity regardless of the hellish reality in which we find those who are marginalized.

Persistent Withdrawal

If the person still refuses to participate,

- Make the task easier and highlight your valuing for any approximation toward participation.
- Avoid getting into a tug-of-war with the person; engagement with us is the immediate purpose, not skill acquisition.
- Give the person some breathing room. Do not rush.
- Be prepared to patiently do this for a while knowing that almost all participation and valuing interactions are dependent upon you.
- Go to where the person is instead of expecting the individual to come to you.

There is a multitude of re-engagement strategies. You might have to bring participation about on the floor or on a sidewalk. It depends on where the person is. We need to stay a step ahead and enable participation at any level. In each situation, we have to remember that the direction of our efforts needs to begin with and lead to increased valuing. Thus, we need to be ready to constantly change our procedures. At one moment it might be helpful to provide gestural cues, at another moment physical assistance. It may be necessary to go to another room or even outside if the person runs away. Teaching can and should occur wherever necessary.

Running Away

If the person runs from the classroom, workplace, or home into a potentially dangerous situation,

- Quickly catch up with the person in as inconspicuous a manner as possible without making it seem like a hunt.
- Attempt to slow down further progress, unless this would result in a physical confrontation, by engaging the person in an activity such as "Let's sit down on the bench over there," "Let's go for a walk," "Let's look at . . .," "Give me a handshake." Continue giving valuing.
- If possible, physically value the person through holding hands.
- As soon as the person's urge to run subsides, try to get him or her to return to the appropriate place.
- Establish a concrete goal such as "I will help you do five, then we will take a break."
- The next time, go on a "break" before the person flees.
- At the worst moments, be the kindest and most nurturing.

Many individuals run away from what they perceive as unpleasant or meaningless situations. So we need to make sure that we represent something good to the individual. Other marginalized persons run away when they are denied access to something they like. For example, if a person insists on having coffee and the caregiver refuses to provide it, this might result in the person bolting for the coffee pot. It is often better to allow the person to have what they desire. If we "legalize" such desires, they tend to lose their power. In addition, as we make these compromises, we should accompany the person and continue to give valuing while drinking coffee. In essence, we permit that which is forbidden and at the same time continue to engage the person in a task in order to teach that engagement is more meaningful than the attention given to "rule" breaking. The temporary legalization of a "forbidden" behavior (e.g., coffee, music, smoking) helps to designify it.

Throwing Objects

If the person throws objects,

- Prevent it by improving environmental arrangements.
- For awhile, manage the materials that are being used instead of tempting the person to throw them.
- Proceed with the task, ignoring the thrown objects on the floor.
- Do not feel compelled to make the person pick them up.
- Do not use punishment consequences, such as overcorrection, restitution, and the like.
- Create a spirit of dialogue in spite of the flung objects.

We frequently feel compelled to immediately correct misdeeds. However, we want to give a new meaning to being with us. Compliance and orderliness are not the goals; companionship is. If a person throws objects, he or she is telling us that there is no joy in the task or that there is more value in doing something else, even being punished. All of our efforts need to lead to valuing, not correction, restraint, or punishment. The need to correct is our need. It is more preferable to continue to teach participation.

Throwing Up

If the person throws up food and reswallows it or spits it out,

- Understand that such self-stimulation tells us about how the person perceives those around him or her. It is a strong message that our presence is less meaningful than swallowing vomit.
- Say nothing about the behavior, but increase valuing, especially physical interactions to clearly indicate that human touch can be good.
- Keep on bringing about participation and make sure that any physical help is nondemanding.

- Watch the seating arrangement to avoid being spat upon.
- If you become soiled, say nothing, keep a towel handy to clean yourself, and continue participation and valuing.
- Consult a physician to make sure there are no physical causes or side effects.

Rumination, regurgitation, and projectile vomiting are significant forms of self-stimulatory behaviors that develop into self-injury. Their underlying causes are many. It is sad when an individual finds more joy in life through self-induced vomiting than in human interactions. We need to be careful to use our physical interactions for tactile valuing and intensely teach the person that our touch is inherently more meaningful than vomiting. This will be a difficult process since self-stimulatory behaviors become entrenched habits. Even as the person becomes engaged and accepting, we still need to deal with the occasional reappearances of the behavior. The more intense our engagement and the warmer our valuing, the more likely we will be able to diminish the habit.

Eating Dangerous Objects

If the person tries to eat dangerous objects like paper clips, gravel, or cigarette butts (i.e., pica),

- Be cautious and prevent harm through environmental arrangements, but still use ordinary settings.
- When presenting tasks, initially shadow the person's hand movements to block the possibility of putting objects in the mouth.
- Emphasize tactile valuing.
- Gradually make the environment more complex.
- Fade these supports as interactional harmony begins to emerge.

This is another form of self-stimulatory and self-injurious behavior. The person may lunge toward dangerous objects and try to ingest harmful substances. This behavior draws caregivers toward the person for restraint. Our punishing can easily become valuing to the person because he or she learns that there is more stimulation and attention given to the behavior than to human interactions. We need to replace this misguided learning with the meaning of valuing in human interactions. A highly structured day is critical since this behavior, like the previous one, is a clear sign that the person's world is empty of consistently warm interactions.

Over the years, individuals learn to withdraw into a primitive world when no hands are reaching toward them. The withdrawn person just sits and stares. And, for example, unable to initiate value-centered interactions, the person might reach to the floor and lick whatever is lying there. At this moment, caregivers will likely yell and grab at him. The person thinks, "Well, this attention is better than nothing." The behavior thus worsens and caregiver reactions become more punishing.

Self-Injury

If the person engages in self-injurious behaviors such as head banging or eye gouging,

- Eliminate the use of helmets, masks, straitjackets, and other forms of restraint.
- Increase staffing to a one-to-one ratio.
- Be prepared to provide intense caregiving for several days to weeks.
- Use flexible environmental arrangement strategies and position yourself and the person, without the use of restraint, in order to prevent self-injury. If necessary, move the person away from walls, table tops, arms of chairs, and other hard or protruding surfaces.
- Gently redirect the person to the task when he or she begins to lash out.
- If this causes a tug-of-war, shadow the blows, allowing the person to strike your hand or arm instead of him- or herself.

- Remember your task and commitment at any given moment is threefold: protect, enable participation, and give valuing.
- Dialogue while gesturally or physically redirecting and protecting.
- Gradually fade the supported environmental arrangements as the behavior decreases in intensity and as calmness emerges.

Self-injurious behavior can bring out the worst or the best in us. The worst, for example, is the use of cattle prods, a commonly reported technique. It is a paradox that punishment is the recommended treatment of choice for those who only find joy in hurting themselves. If we are to be congruent with our beliefs and values, our focus needs to be on enabling the individual to engage with us and others so that he or she can learn the meaning of our presence, words, and touch. This requires teaching intensity, the prevention of harm, the sensitive timing of warm assistance, and ongoing dialogue. We need to express deep empathy, understand the profound and anguished despair inherent in this harm, and help the person resignify the meaning of the human condition. Practically speaking, our arms and hands need to become the protectors. We need to position ourselves so as to be able to both enable participation and block or shadow attempts at injury. Our pace of interactions should be steady and smooth, avoiding even momentary interruptions. Since we are using a large amount of physical blocking, we need to dramatically increase our physical valuing so that the person learns that we represent valuing.

Disorganized Verbal Expressions

If the person talks incessantly or inappropriately or screams,

- Say nothing about the inappropriateness of what is being said.

- Listen carefully and focus your attention on the kernels of truth in the disorganized thoughts and use these as themes for your dialogue.
- Give value for participation, even though the person might continue to talk or scream.
- Involve the person in a mutual conversation, initiating and structuring it so that the person expresses more meaningful and connected communication.
- Use this as another vehicle to value the person.

Many caregivers tell the person to be silent, verbally punish the person, or make fun of the person. Others try to use cognitive therapy and reason out the disorganized thought. Inappropriate conversation is similar to other disruptive behaviors that require learning of the meaning of dialogue. It is important to redirect the person toward participatory interactions, whether through words or deeds. It might be necessary to accept and go along with the "silly" conversation for a few moments, but remembering what might seem silly to us is important to the person. The challenge is to bring it into a shared reality. In the beginning, our dialogue will be parallel with the person's vocalizations. Our role is to weave the dialogue in and out of the person's stream of thought and gradually merge our feelings with theirs.

If the conversation is a symptom of a mental illness such as schizophrenia, we need to focus on establishing a flow of thought congruent with the here-and-now and highlight their engagement with us. This has nothing to do with the shallowness of reality therapy, but rather involves centering the person on what it means to be with us, to be valued by us, and to reciprocate this valuing.

We need to listen carefully to what the person is expressing. Seedlings of truth exist in hallucinations: fear, joy, hope, and despair. These can become themes in our dialogue. Even if the disorganized thought is due to a psychosis, there is no reason why we cannot teach increasingly more reality-based patterns of thoughts and feelings through dialogue, while at the same time respecting the person.

Depression

If the person is depressed,

- Be especially warm in all interactions.
- Create an external emotional structure by intensifying and increasing human contact throughout the day.
- Dramatically increase verbal and tactile valuing in a way that emphasizes your enduring desire to be with the person.
- Take advantage of physical assistance as a way to soothe and reassure the person.
- Understand and deal with the causes of the depression, but also help reintroduce new meaning into the individual's life.
- Examine the support structure around the person and help re-establish a network of friends capable of meeting the person's needs.

As devastating as depression is, it nevertheless points to the full sentient nature of the person, a point often forgotten. Like everyone else, marginalized people can become depressed due to loss and the inability to reach out. Indeed, their vulnerabilities make their depression more likely. All people hunger for being with others. When this need is unfulfilled, the individual is emptied of life's meaning and drowns in a choiceless world. We need to represent the rebirth of hope. It is important to show tolerance, affection, and warmth; in effect, we temporarily become the person's emotional support and lead the person out of depression. As we do this, we need to ensure the formation of a circle of friends who will reach out to the person.

Custodial Settings

If you think your work is in the poorest setting in the world and that interdependence is impossible,

- Initially focus on the needs of the persons whom you serve, not the entire system.

- Prioritize the individuals according to who has the severest need to receive valuing.
- Be with that person whatever the number of minutes per day in order to at least begin to touch on his or her's longing for relatedness.
- Make sure the person is actively involved.
- Envision the most difficult person as able to bond with you.
- Over time, publicly advocate for systemic change.
- Organize residents, other caregivers, parents, and community members to bring about social change.

Although there are horrendous settings in which hundreds of thousands of persons live around the world, one caregiver can begin to make a difference. If we work in solidarity with each other, then it is quite possible to change oppressive environments. If we enter into alliances with others, such as parent advocacy organizations and labor unions, then substantive change is that much more likely. Even the caregiver with the most humble job should be aware that his or her work is a community act that requires constant reflection and action. Union advocates especially have a dramatic and powerful role in improving or changing the quality of life of union members and the persons whom they serve. A posture of solidarity should be evident in the ongoing struggle of organized workers, especially if the welfare of the workers is clearly perceived as being intertwined with the welfare of marginalized people. Those who work in institutions are challenged to bring warmth where frigidity reigns. Those who work among the homeless are asked to bring safety and security in the back alleys of city streets. Those who toil in slums are called on to bring hope where there is despair.

Pro-Punishment

When other caregivers want to use punishment,

- Show the seriousness of your intention to avoid punishment through your personal advocacy.

- Notify an outside advocate of the use of the punishment or restraint.
- Refuse to agree to such interventions.
- Demonstrate on your own a value-centered approach.
- Persevere and become politically active with the intent of helping to create new laws and procedures that enhance the quality of life rather than diminish it.
- Initiate lawsuits to protect human rights.

Interdisciplinary teams came into being to enhance and broaden the decision-making process and protect human rights. However, they are often groups of professionals who legitimize and rubber-stamp inadequate services or even human rights violations. Procedural correctness often replaces human rights. We need to work together and realize that the primary questions revolve around values and how these influence what we do and how we do it. For an interdisciplinary team to validate the use of punishment and restraint makes human wrongs into human rights. The end does not justify the means. Rather, we need to opt for interdependence through the just means of unconditional valuing. We need to actively pursue the goals of bonding and interdependence and speak out when these become replaced by compliance and submission. Most importantly, we need to demonstrate our values in our daily actions.

Psychoactive Drugs

If the person is taking psychoactive medications,

- With the supervision of a psychiatrist, see what the person is like medication-free.
- Make sure the drug is based on a meaningful diagnosis.
- Engage the person in an active daily program to see what the individual is like and to determine the need for drugs.
- Avoid the use of drugs for singular behavioral problems such as aggression.

- If helpful, use drugs to initially enable the person to be more available and responsive to being with you and others.
- If used, reduce the dosage as the person moves toward friendship.
- Eliminate the use of drugs as soon as possible.

Psychoactive drugs can sometimes be therapeutic when a person has a mental illness such as schizophrenia or manic depression. However, it is unethical to use drugs simply to control behaviors. Chemical restraint is the modern alternative to straitjackets. It arises out of the same authoritarian posture. Even when drugs are necessary to treat an underlying mental illness, they should be used with care, discretion, and the intent to decrease or eliminate their use. We need to work with psychiatrists and sensitize one another. Drugs are only one therapeutic option. We need to ensure the exploration of alternatives and make certain that the drugs are not a substitute for decent places to live or a replacement for caregiving.

Lack of Success

If nothing has seemed to work,

- Examine your values, your commitment, and the culture in which you are working.
- Ask yourself whether you are focusing on the task or the interaction and whether the "system" is dehumanizing or not.
- Question whether you are expressing a sufficiently high degree of valuing and human engagement. Remember what you might think is enough valuing is often quite insufficient.
- Examine the degree of warm help that you are giving to the person and the frequency and timing of your valuing.
- Reflect on the spirit of dialogue that exists in your interactions.

Many persons are extremely challenging to help. If caregivers bring a history of punishment or restraint to their interactions with the person, it is difficult to transform this posture. Some places and situations are nothing more than jails with jailkeepers instead of caregivers. Although we often feel that we are sufficiently valuing a person, it is helpful to step back and analyze the types of interactions that occur in day-to-day life. We may be ignoring the person instead of the behavior, confronting the person instead of re-engaging, or prompting and correcting the person rather than valuing. At times we have poor timing. We value the deed done instead of the person. We see precursors to outbursts, but delay our intervention and worsen the problem. Often, we deliver reward instead of unconditionally valuing the person. We need to look at ourselves, those around us, and the world in which we work. Change has to occur at all these levels.

Fighting

If one person fights with another,

- Give the necessary assistance to the person attacked and make sure adequate protection is available.
- Recenter yourself on the person who committed the aggression, engage the individual in an activity, and establish this and valuing as the core of their life condition.
- Avoid future attacks through better environmental management, more sensitive redirection before violence occurs, and an analysis of the degree of support that each person requires.
- Engage each in participatory interactions in order to teach mutuality and sharing.
- Avoid verbal or physical reprimands.

Violence rarely occurs without warning signs. Frustration, lack of communication skills, lack of life meaning, poor groupings of persons, boredom, caregiver inattentiveness, plus a multitude of other reasons can cause aggression. Once it happens, we need to analyze these variables and restructure the environment and interactions accordingly. The first rule of caregiving is that harm comes to no one, but once aggression occurs, our focus has to be on engagement and valuing. We do not need to teach the aggressor a lesson through punishment. The challenge is to resignify what it means to interact and then teach the aggressor and the attacked to learn to live together.

Severe Mental Retardation

If the person fails to respond at all or minimally,

- Give warm help. Work hand-over-hand if the person is not fearful of this.
- Avoid getting into a tug-of-war if the person refuses even warm help.
- Instead of physically helping someone, place an activity in his or her hand.
- Use your touch for valuing.
- Simplify the task to ensure success.
- Use errorless teaching techniques to help the person participate without frustration.
- Seek tasks that are within the person's ability.
- Teach an alternate means of communication such as gestures or signing.
- Gradually fade assistance so that overdependence is avoided.

Regardless of the person's actual or supposed ability, we have the responsibility for enabling participation so that valuing can be linked to the feeling of being together. A major challenge is to create a structure that brings us together with the person and serves as a vehicle for engagement and valuing. Severe mental retardation leaves the individual vulnerable to self-isolation. It makes it harder for the person to communicate with others. Our responsibility is to literally teach reaching out to others. We have to put aside our compulsion to make people independent. Instead, our role is to nurture human development, accept the wholeness of the individual no matter what, and create a spirit of interdependence.

Age-Inappropriateness

If the person interacts with you or others age-inappropriately,

- Value adult-like interactions, but encourage playfulness and friendliness.
- If the person is hugging excessively, slowly change this to handshakes or pats on the back.
- Engage the person in an activity and include these particular interactions in the flow of the day.
- Make certain that other caregivers utilize and emphasize learning adult-like interactions.
- Avoid a posture of overprotection.

Some persons feel that interactions that physically value an individual, such as hugs, can produce age-inappropriate behaviors. However, this will not occur if we focus on the appropriateness of the interactions. The question is not so much whether these are good or bad, but when, where, and to what degree they occur. To give a strong indication of unconditional valuing, as well as feelings of security, it is helpful to physically value the person, especially at the start of the change process. Indeed, instead of these exaggerated interactions, what occurs more frequently is the lack of warm human interactions. Many persons learn inappropriate ways of interacting because they hunger for human warmth and affection, yet receive little or none. Physical valuing can serve as a strong and concrete expression of solidarity during the initial dimensions of the mutual change process. After a few hours or days, we can then transform these into more common value-centered interactions.

Group Home

If you feel that there is not enough time to teach friendship and companionship in your group home,

- Make sure your home is a true home: small, personalized, and family centered.
- Look at the natural flow of the day and increase the number of opportunities to come together.
- Understand that much of the home's routine can become a series of opportunities to give valuing, offer warm help, and teach sharing.
- Focus on self-care skills and daily living skills as vehicles for valuing.
- Look at your role as one of a family member rather than as a staff person.
- For more challenging individuals, structure situations so that intense opportunities for interdependence are constantly available.
- Use the insight and practical techniques that you learn in these more structured times as the basis for your techniques in less-structured times and settings.

Group homes are places for learning to live together. They are not just facilities that provide room and board, but rather their central purpose is to nurture feelings of family, interdependence, and community. They need to express family life, community, and the togetherness. Of course, this spirit becomes more difficult to create in settings where an excessive number of people are grouped or where everyone has similar problems. Sharing is not expected or taught. There is a multitude of practical and necessary activities in the home that can serve as vehicles for teaching valuing, such as self-care and daily living skills. These need to be structured into the person's day as a means to bring about participation and facilitate unconditional valuing. Group living often ends up to be custodial care with each individual living parallel to the other. Names are not known. Feelings are not respected. Each is an island. Such places establish a modicum of control through dispensing tokens for obedience. However, we are challenged to focus on relationships and the establishment of family feelings by bringing people together.

Danger to Self or Others

If the person is termed as a danger to self or others due to antisocial behavior,

- Structure the person's day, regardless of their "functioning level."
- Consider that cognitive ability has little to do with emotional connectedness.
- Avoid any focus on "I have to teach this person a lesson!"
- Give adequate supervision to the person and ensure community protection.
- Give ample valuing and opportunities for dialogue with an emphasis on respect for others and rules for living.
- Expect to provide such structure and supervision for a considerable period of time.

One of the most challenging groups to serve is one of persons who have infrequent but devastating behaviors, such as child molestation. They are often in and out of the criminal justice system and pass through a myriad of foster homes with no stability. They require long-term support and guidance, but often live in unstable and poorly structured settings. A misleading perception exists that equates cognitive ability with emotional stability. Caregivers often think that if they increase their help they are being manipulated or if they increase structure and supervision they are denying right. It is often heard, "Well, he should know better!" The fact is the person does not and is stuck in an emotional quagmire. Also, we have a grave responsibility to protect the community from destructive acts against others. Even though persons with these needs generally have multiple skills, it is necessary to structure and supervise their lives. This can often be accomplished in a small group home or supported foster home setting. But any setting has to guarantee the community that harm will come to nobody. It is critical to remember that people with these needs will probably need maximum support across their life spans, regardless of their "functioning" level. The basic elements of this structure are ongoing supervision and enabling the person to formulate and practice just rules for living. The rules for living are accomplished through ongoing dialogue. This needs to be concrete, other-centered, and modeled in reality. The person has to learn what respectful relationships consist of, and this can only be accomplished through ongoing structure, supervision, and guidance.

Exploitation

If the person is being exploited,

- Focus first on attempting to delineate whether the person is aware of the exploitation.
- Concretely explain the nature of the exploitation.
- Analyze the degree of residential support the person requires: a live-in staff person for a time, return to a group home for more significant structure, or more consistent case advocacy.
- Counsel the individual over time regarding what exploitation and fairness are through role-modeling and multiple positive experiences.
- Make sure the person has someone to give guidance and support.

There is a delicate balance between dependence and independence. Many with mental retardation or chronic mental illness are reared and educated in protective settings and when "given" independence, they are poorly prepared for it. Many persons require significantly more emotional support than their "functioning skills" might indicate. The goal is interdependence. Also, children and adults in dysfunctional families or programs are vulnerable to rebel against authority or the lack of affection by becoming targets of exploitation. We need to be sensitive to this and be ready to provide guidance.

Counseling

If you are involved in counseling,

- Clarify the purpose of each session.
- Engage the person in dialogue that reflects feelings, delineates hope, removes despair or confusion, and guides the person toward the formation of interdependent relationships.
- Express warmth and authenticity.
- Help define problems and select choices.
- Help identify and mobilize a network of support and a circle of friends.
- Help center a person.
- Focus on concrete topics and options that will help bring the person into reality.

We need to listen closely and dialogue. However, we can fall into the trap of giving undue attention to problematic behaviors. We need to recognize this and help individuals reflect on them from the perspective of just relationships. A major element is to support the person emotionally and to guide them directly through difficult times. We are their model. Our primary task is to instill hope. We need to understand and empathize with the person's history and reality. The underlying theme is to help the individual move through a process of becoming other-centered. It is important to avoid a primary focus on behavior problems and create feelings of union solely with us, and then help the person find ways to integrate this into their daily lives. Our tone needs to be kind and warm. We have to perceive the person's fears and anguish. Counseling is a coming together over time. We are often the person's only friend in the beginning, and our first purpose is to reveal this and then spread it outwardly.

The individual will often be unable to articulate personal feelings except through distancing behaviors. As we initiate dialogue, it is helpful to share our own joys and sorrows while also helping the person see options. Since loneliness is a frequent travel mate of marginalized people, it is critical that we explore the degree of community support that the person has. This often involves bringing significant others into the counseling process and helping them commit themselves to ongoing friendship. Sometimes this circle of friends does not exist or is insufficient, and so we need to help establish a support network. Throughout the process, our dialogue needs to focus on themes that relate to interdependence. This requires concreteness and the definition of abstract feelings. The person who has no friends does not know what friendship is. The person who is in despair does not know what hope is. We need to model such feelings and help the person develop alternative ways to establish them.

Relating with Others in Counseling

If you are having trouble relating to the person,

- Focus on the individual as a companion.
- Recognize human anguish, not just observable behaviors.
- Recenter the person toward feelings of solidarity.
- Help turn the person's gaze away from self and toward others.
- Share the meaning of your life with the person.
- Help remove obstacles to human engagement.
- Use your own self and your personal history as a model for personal commitment and identity.

We have to know ourselves before we reach out to others. If we find little meaning in life, it is impossible to reveal it in others. If we are selfish, it is impossible to encourage companionship in others. If we are oppressors, it is impossible to help free others. As we deepen our understanding of our own life's meaning, we can better recognize and deal with the other person's profound and pervasive mind-set. This involves a refocusing process and a critical questioning of our and the other's beliefs and values. It will often be necessary to deflect aggressive or avoidant expressions by helping the person turn his or her gaze from selfishness to "otherness" and from ambiguity to concreteness. The central purpose in establishing a relationship is to effectuate engagement with others. This involves a feeling of being in union with others, caring about others, and using one's talents to reach out to and share with others. Through this process, we need to recognize that we are a model for personal commitment and identity. What the person sees in us serves to instill hope if our interactions are centered on dialogue.

Experiences in Mutual Change

"What do you do if . . . ?" questions can be asked and answered in an infinite number of ways. Each person's uniqueness tells us that there are no fixed answers; rather, the common ground is a shared purpose and process. Our strategies and techniques need to be based on enabling engagement and unconditional valuing. We and the marginalized person bring a history to the emerging relationship. Each has talents and needs. The central rule is value-centeredness, and it is on this that all our decisions need to be made. The key question, then, is always, "Is what I am doing valuing the other?" It is critical to avoid the entrapment of "Will it result in valuing?" since this would make our interactions contingent upon "good" behavior. By then, it would be too late and too mechanistic. No matter what specific techniques we might consider, our challenge is to constantly measure our interactions with the yard stick of valuing.

Our experiences in attempting to become more value-centered and to express dialogue have required us to flexibly use supportive techniques in the designify–resignify process. Always trying to center ourselves on unconditional valuing, the challenge then is how to designify violence and bring feelings of companionship in specific life situations. Several case histories will hopefully provide some insight into the unique process that each individual presents. These examples are only a brief slice out of each person's life and are presented to give an idea of the moment-to-moment decision-making that we go through as we strive to establish new meanings in our relationship.

Georgie

Georgie was a 9-year-old child who attended a local school and lived with his parents and two younger brothers. He had a history of self-injury for six years, as well as active withdrawal from interactions. His parents were lovingly involved in his life, although perplexed by his self-injury. He was unable to verbally communicate. He had a diagnosis of cerebral palsy and severe mental retardation. He was also nonambulatory and spent a considerable amount of time with his arms and lap tied to his wheelchair. His parents and teacher had resorted to the use of restraints as the only way they could protect him from harm. He sometimes enjoyed having others nearby, but he only knew how to gain attention through his head-banging or tossing items onto the floor. His caregivers generally gave into his wishes and he seemed to have learned to engage in these behaviors to draw people toward himself, even if that were to result in reprimands or restraints. Past intervention strategies had included the use of gloves on his hands to control his self-hitting, holding him down, time-out, and verbal reprimands. He also usually received verbal praise and a token when he was compliant. However, once removed from restraint, he often engaged in punching his nose, slapping his face, or slamming his head to his arms. In spite of these behaviors, when given attention, he could be quite playful and enjoyed laughing with his caregivers or at the difficulties that he presented to them.

Whenever his teacher freed him from restraint, he spent most of the time scooting away from her. If she tried to engage him on a task, he would swat the materials away and laugh. When she decreased her attention toward him, he would lift his arm up and try to slap his face or bite his hand. Unfortunately, as often happens, she would switch from one activity to another in an attempt to find something that he might be interested in. She did not realize that the task was not the issue, but rather his perception of her. Although he would momentarily participate, he inevitably would become disinterested in a few moments and would move away. If she did not find another task, he would become overly anxious and hit himself several times. Thus, Georgie presented several challenges to his caregivers: self-injury, inattentiveness, a history of restraint and punishment, and little consistency in the expression of feelings of companionship.

When his teacher resolved to enter into a mutual change process with him, she first sat beside him to help bring about participation on a simple task. It was not necessary to be too concerned about his self-injury since he was slow and she could protect him in time by placing her hands between his hand and his face. Since he enjoyed attention, she decided to concentrate on bringing about engagement and linking that with unconditional valuing. She used errorless teaching techniques and essentially forgot about his ability to do the task and focused on ensuring a smooth flow of mutual participation. Her purpose was to teach him that she was a constant source of valuing and that doing tasks together was a vehicle for this. After several hours, she placed him in a regular chair since it was important to take away distancing meanings such as those represented by the restraint chair. His need to be restrained and to be in that particular chair separated him from others. Straps had replaced kind touch. She was careful to sit next to him in such a way so as to be able to protect him whenever he tried to hit himself. Because she gave ongoing valuing, he did not give much indication of anger or uneasiness and continued to participate well. He stayed in the chair the rest of the day and even started to reach out toward her instead of trying to slap himself.

In these first hours, the teacher had to deal with multiple challenges. When freeing him from restraint, she had to use her hands and arms to block his attempts at self-injury. When placing him in an ordinary chair, she had to deal with his cries for his restraint chair. When using a task, she had to prevent him from throwing the materials. When he refused to participate, she had to find ways to enable it. When he was not responding to her valuing, she had to intensify and personalize it. The teacher became involved in a swirl of movements; one hand helping, the other protecting; one moment placing one of the task materials in his hand, the next helping him do the task; one moment patting him on the back, the next doing the task with him to ensure a flow to the participation. Within all of this, she had to quickly learn how to value him unconditionally, sometimes emphasizing his initiation of minimal participation: "Wow! You are doing this all by yourself!"; sometimes highlighting their togetherness: "Look at us! We are doing this like two friends!"; sometimes disregarding objects tossed on the floor: "I am sorry! I will give you more help. Friends do this kind of work together." She had to learn to center herself on participation and valuing in an ebb and flow: sometimes giving more help, sometimes less; sometimes slowing down, sometimes speeding up; sometimes pointing out their friendship, sometimes valuing his participation.

As she became more comfortable and adept, and as Georgie began to participate more, she decided to expand their emerging relationship to other children. She noticed two other boys who seemed interested. She invited them to help her teach Georgie to share—to be with other children, to do a task together, and to show their friendship. She brought them together, sat between them, and orchestrated a joint task. In the beginning, she was almost Georgie's hands and voice, helping him every step of the way: "Okay, Georgie, all four of us are going to learn to do things together. I will give you all the help you need." Her hands worked with Georgie's as they handed one of the materials to one of the boys. Georgie tried to scoot it away, but she continued the movement while saying, "Look at what we are doing! These kids know how to help each other just like us. Here it goes in Jim's hand. And now, let's not forget the most important thing, a handshake!" The other boys enjoyed the process and waited for Georgie's reluctant participation. They began to help him in the same way as the teacher. Soon, they were giving unconditional valuing as well. Georgie began to smile, wait his turn, and do more on his own. Thus began the progressive movement toward human interdependence—slowly, surely, and inevitably.

What do George and his teacher show us? In a few days, Georgie had moved from self-centered behaviors to the beginning of other-centered ones. He was starting to learn that his teacher was a source of valuing and that it was good to be with others. This process took time and effort. We have to be willing to tolerate initial difficulty and create ways to prevent harm. Although we have a clear duty to protect, this does not have to equate with restraint. It can involve making sure that we sit or stand by the person so we can raise our hands to let blows strike us. Even more importantly, it requires a focus on prevention. In the beginning, this means that we have to take the time to give sufficient attention to the person and help develop the feeling that participation with us is good. If Georgie is tied up, he cannot learn; if we are too busy, we cannot teach. It was hard for the teacher to find the time to be with Georgie. Yet, she knew that she had to dedicate extra effort if she were to help him develop a feeling of friendship. This is no easy task for caregivers since the first hours or days can be quite frustrating. We might try one thing to protect the person and it does not work. Then we try another and another. We can easily throw our hands up and give up. Georgie's teacher was willing to endure these initial frustrations and search for non-punishing ways to protect him and enable participation. Another problem is that we can become so involved in one aspect of caregiving, such as protection, that we forget about participation or the expression of unconditional valuing. Georgie's teacher had to learn to use her whole being: one hand protecting, the other bringing about participation; at one moment scooting materials aside, at the next patting him on the back; at one moment her words consoling him, and at the next encouraging him. This took considerable energy, concentration, and creativity. If she had focused on decreasing his behavioral problems, she would not have been able to establish the beginning of a new meaning to their relationship. Freeing him from restraint and protecting him was a necessary prelude to the resignification process.

John

John was a 35-year-old man with mild mental retardation and autism, with a number of withdrawn, self-injurious, and aggressive behaviors. He had been institutionalized most of his life and was currently residing in a community residence with one other person with a mental handicap. He was a very driven person, having little tolerance of others, fearful of them, and anxious to remove himself from human contact. He spent most of his time alone and would swat away anyone who approached him, or would simply run to a distant corner where he would continue his self-stimulation. He spent much time pacing back and forth, moaning, lifting up his shirt, biting his fingernails, and flapping his arms. When anyone asked him to participate in an activity, he would typically push them forcefully, yell, and, if they persisted, he would strike out, scratch, and attempt to choke them. He was unwilling to participate in any task and preferred to jump up and search for coffee or toss any objects that were within his reach. When angry, he would begin rubbing his eyes; as his consternation increased, he would dig his fists into his eye sockets. The only activities that he was interested in were spending long periods of time by himself and drinking coffee. He lived a solitary life in a sorrowful condition. His caregivers were frustrated by the intensity and distancing nature of his interactions as well as his underlying fear, his rejection of affection and human warmth, and his propensity to enter into a state of self-isolation. They preferred to leave him alone since any requests would lead to violence.

When a caregiver resolved to enter into a mutual change process with John, he decided to "legalize" his strong desire for coffee since John would inevitably fight for it. In the first attempts, John refused to sit, stand still, or accept any valuing. His gaze moved from one object to another. He made no meaningful eye contact. When physically valued or helped, he pushed the caregiver away. He rushed from one location to another seeking coffee since he had consumed all that had been made for him. He scavenged through materials and trash cans and tossed objects onto the floor. The caregiver, seeing the intensity of his interactions, resolved to accompany him and bring about any level of participation and to link this with a dialogue regarding friendship and doing things together. This was much easier said than done. For John, the caregiver's presence triggered violence. The caregiver had to learn to stay with him, engage in dialogue, and do activities with and for him, even while on the move. He gave him ongoing valuing through words and actions and kept up with him. John initially paid no heed to his words and kept avoiding any physical contact. Nevertheless, the caregiver persisted and John occasionally seemed to accept the valuing since he would look now and then and even place his hand momentarily in the caregiver's. He also began to slightly increase his participation on the activity and tolerated the caregiver's brief interactions. However, within moments, he would invariably jump up, push the caregiver aside, and bolt away.

On one occasion, he attacked the caregiver, digging his fingernails into his neck and arms. The caregiver designified this by not responding, remaining warm, and continuing to express value. He continued to enable participation and simultaneously carried on a dialogue. John attempted to injure himself several times by trying to forcefully rub his fists in his eyes. The caregiver resignified those interactions by placing his arm to block these attempts while also continuing to engage him on a particular task. These first hours were extremely difficult for John and the caregiver. Nothing made sense to John. The caregiver had to remain calm, enable participation, and express valuing.

As the hours unfolded, John gradually participated more and decreased the intensity of his aggression, withdrawal, and attempts at self-injury. He started to linger for longer periods of time with his caregiver and accept handshakes, embraces, and verbal valuing. He also began to initiate some reciprocation of valuing through slight smiles, gazes, and, eventually, embraces and handshakes. His moaning and yelling began to turn to soothing sounds.

Within two weeks, his aggression had disappeared with this particular caregiver. Rather than running away, he accepted invitations to take short walks and willingly returned to the activity.

What do John and his caregiver teach us? An important thing to remember is to stay calm and collected at the most frustrating moments. When he was digging his fingernails into the caregiver's arm, it would have been common for the caregiver to become angry and retaliatory—all in the name of behavioral control. We often hear comments such as, "We cannot let him get away with that!" Yet, once the behavior has occurred, the challenge is to resignify what the relationship means and prevent future aggression. When he refused to come with the caregiver and do his activity, it would have been typical to "escort" him to his place. During these times, we have to remember that our central strategy is to give valuing. A person's refusal to participate often irritates caregivers and gives rise to the desire to control in a "My God, he has got to obey!" feeling. This has to be checked and turned into a process of going to where the person is, moving with the individual, staying a step ahead, and continuing any mutual involvement. However, we often fail to accompany the person and expect the individual to come to us. This is like watching someone drown instead of reaching out to save them. It is also important to remember to elicit valuing by extending our hand to the person, touching or seeking any sort of physical contact, even when it is rejected. Once the valuing process takes root, distancing interactions begin to diminish and change. Running away becomes less frequent, less long-lasting, and less intense. As this occurs, the caregiver, then, has a much better chance of increasing engagement and expanding it to others.

Claudette

Claudette was a 28-year-old woman with a diagnosis of schizophrenia and a long history of life-threatening self-injurious behaviors that included head-banging on floors and walls; pinching and scratching her face, arms, and legs; slapping her face; and pulling her hair out. She also had a range of aggressive interactions that included hitting, slapping, pinching, and pulling hair. She engaged in disruptive behaviors such as throwing tables and tipping over chairs. She had several other interactions related to withdrawing from human contact, such as sliding onto the floor and scooting and crawling away whenever anyone came near her. She had basic self-care skills and was verbal. She had adequate receptive and expressive language, but tended to communicate through her behaviors rather than her words. Claudette had resided in a public institution most of her adult life, but had spent a brief period of time in a community residential setting when she was 25 years old. However, she was readmitted to the institution after a few months due to her self-injury and aggression. It had been assumed that the mere act of deinstitutionalization and community placement would bring an end to her severe difficulties. Yet, this did not result in any behavioral amelioration since those caregivers were unable or unwilling to cope with her and continued to focus on compliance.

Her body was stigmatized by multiple scars and wounds from her self-injury: Her forehead had a large circular wound with fresh blood; her face bore over a dozen deep scratches on both cheeks, her nose, and lips; and her left leg also had a deep wound from gouging her skin. Most unfortunately, she was blind in both eyes due to detached retinas produced by her head-banging. She presented a very sad and anguished countenance and seemed driven by anger. She screamed and demanded solitude. Her caregivers generally had to "escort" her from place to place. Her violence was almost always met by their violence. They appeared tired and frustrated by her intense attempts at aggression and self-injury and their inability to gain what they desired: control.

Previous interventions had included attempts at positive reinforcement. But the preponderance of past treatment had involved the use of various forms of punishment and restraint since contingent reward was meaningless to her: overcorrection, time

out, physical holds, mechanical devices such as a straitjacket, psychoactive medications, and a number of other behavioral control
approaches. Her most recent intervention had been the use of a
locked seclusion room where she was placed for up to ten hours
per day with minimal supervision. Although she was supposed to
receive on-going monitoring, she often gouged her face, hands,
and arms in this lonely room.

When one of her caregivers resolved to enter a mutual change
process with Claudette, it was difficult to enable her to participate.
She generally preferred to scoot or move about the room and
would swat him away when attempts were made to resignify their
interactions as value-centered rather than dominative. Her attempts at self-injury required ongoing alertness, and her caregiver
had to be ready to block her hits, always without grabbing her. It
was important to speak softly and soothingly since loudness led to
more intensely driven behavior. Because of her tactile defensiveness and her blindness, it was quite difficult to bring about participation. She feared being touched. If the caregiver took her by
the hand, she would jerk away. To facilitate participation, he
slipped objects into her hands and made sure that all touch was
warm and valuing. He did not want to convey a feeling of being
demanding. Although she was reluctant at the start to accept any
physical valuing or even stay near the caregiver, she gradually
appeared slightly attentive to his dialogue. He spoke to her about
the meaning of friendship and doing things together while at the
same time continuing the participatory interactions. As this went
on, she occasionally smiled, responded, and reached her hand out
for a handshake several times. These first hours required the caregiver to constantly reflect on his values and put them into practice.
The next day, the first hour was difficult since she again refused to participate and repeatedly said, "No, No, No!" However,
without forcing her, he gradually brought about some minimal
participation by doing most of a task for her. He understood that
an ebb and flow would occur, so he remained focused on participation and dialogue. Over a two-week period, good moments started
to replace aggression and self-injurious ones. Nevertheless, the

caregiver had to be ever-ready to protect her and himself. His interactions became clearer, more concrete, and more centered on their possible relationship. Since she was extremely driven, he had to concentrate on slowing her down by modulating his voice, expressing words and gestures soothingly, and taking many breaks with her. He also had to become quick in his ability to both protect her and enable participation. After two weeks, Claudette displayed no self-injury or aggression. However, she obviously was very vulnerable and fragile. In addition, her relationship with this particular caregiver did not mean that she had developed similar interactions with others. This generalization had to be taught. But, for this caregiver, Claudette was beginning to transmit feelings of companionship: gazes, reaching out, and participating in the dialogue, often with much humor and playfulness. The caregiver was more relaxed and was developing feelings of trust and friendship.

What do Claudette and her caregiver teach us? Her profound anguish calls on us to practice an enduring commitment. Her life-view had been colored by meaninglessness so deep that she had blinded herself and had withdrawn from almost any humanizing engagement. Her blindness and fear of being touched made the process more difficult. It was important to highlight and intensify verbal interactions and make sure that physical contact was demonstrative of warmth and nonviolence. When she needed help to participate, the caregiver had to make sure that he did not give any feeling of force. One way to simplify his help and decrease her perception of being forced to participate was to slip objects into her hand instead of telling her what to do or working hand over hand. Any physical help would have escalated her fear. He needed to learn to avoid touching her hand in any demanding way since caregivers had typically pushed and pulled her over the years. All touch had to communicate warm valuing. Although her self-injury and self-isolation were somewhat similar to Georgie's, it was significantly more intense and dangerous. Claudette's caregiver needed to be constantly on guard and enable engagement and express valuing in the midst of furies. His tone had to be soothing. Every physical movement needed to signal safety. There could not be a hint of control or domination. As their relationship improved, the caregiver sought ways to create a culture of life in a world filled with fear. His emerging companionship with Claudette was only a minute step in a process of mutual and social change.

Maxine

Maxine was a 32-year-old woman who had spent most of her life in a large public institution. In the last year, she had been living in a community residence, but continued to display a range of self-injurious, aggressive, and withdrawn interactional patterns that consisted of biting the top of her hand to the point of breaking her skin, slamming her fist against hard surfaces, punching caregivers forcefully, and wrapping long strings around her left arm stopping blood circulation. Her caregivers avoided taking the string from her arm and described it as her "security blanket." Instead of interacting with others, she preferred to spend her time pacing and alternating between playing with the string and wrapping it tightly around her arm. She had frequent episodes of disorganized speech, especially related to an imaginary police woman who, she reported, was always following her. Her paranoia was quite burdensome and it irritated her caregivers. They told her that the police woman did not exist; yet, this only increased her anxiety. Her behavior intervention program consisted of "verbally reprimanding her for hurting self or others, physically restraining her when biting her hand, removing her from stressful situations, and ignoring her chatter about the police woman." This approach had only served to maintain her aggression, self-injury, and paranoia at a relatively high level—neither increasing it, nor decreasing it. Her caregivers seemed to be satisfied with this stalemate and essentially left her alone, except when harmful interactions emerged. Maxine spent much time in her imaginary world of the police woman. She presented a very lonely appearance. She increasingly rejected human contact, was tactilely defensive, and moved away from others. She seldom smiled and screamed if anyone tried to touch her.

When caregivers tried to work with her, Maxine spent most of the time yelling, "She is coming to get me!" The imagined police woman hovered over her and blocked any meaning in others. She insisted on keeping her arm tightly bound with the string, and caregivers would give this to her as a pacifier. Between the ghost and the string there was little room for caregivers. She showed no warmth or affection in any of her interactions and adamantly refused to be touched even for a handshake or a pat on the back. The more they tried to bring about any participation, the more she would try to bite her hand and pull a piece of skin off it. She would also start to pound the caregiver in the chest with both her fists. She would participate on particular tasks most reluctantly. She did not seem to show any interest in her caregivers' presence, or any form of being valued. Likewise, they seemed disinterested in her.

When a caregiver decided to enter into a mutual change process with Maxine, she began to display many of the same problems. However, this caregiver commenced to give her ongoing valuing in the form of a dialogue about not hurting her or forcing her to do anything; plus, he kept participation occurring, even though he was doing most of the task for her. She initially saw no meaning in any of this, continued to try to bite her hand, lash out, and cry about the police woman. The caregiver blocked her hand whenever it went toward her mouth so as to avoid any harm and, while doing this, also continued to effectuate participation and valuing in spite of her belligerency. When she expressed fear about the police woman, he included the fear in his dialogue, saying, "We are together, I will protect you! Nobody is going to hurt you. That is why it is good to be friends." She began to stay for longer periods of time near the caregiver, and her attempts at self-injury began to decrease. At this point, whenever she walked away, she would stand by herself for a few moments and then return to him. She began to enjoy being with him, but out of habit continued to move away. She started to allow him to touch her hand and then give her a handshake. After several such contacts, he asked her for a hug and she laid her head on his chest and smiled brightly. At this moment, she allowed him to unravel the string from her arm. She became more willing to participate with lessening degrees of help, and every step of the way she waited for a hug or handshake. She would not stay with him for more than a few minutes, yet she was willing to leave, walk away, and then return on her own. As the minutes wore on, these trips became less distant and time-consuming. Her concern about the police woman lessened. After several hours, she did not mention it at all. The dialogue focused more on friendship and Maxine seemed attentive and understanding.

The next day, Maxine participated the entire day without any disruptive interactions—no attempts at self-injury, aggression, or screaming. She mentioned the police woman, but when the caregiver spoke of their friendship, she started to talk about what she would like to do. She sought out and expected physical and verbal valuing. Her tactile defensiveness had become a non-issue. She smiled frequently and vocalized with sounds of happiness. Her countenance had changed. She was relaxed, calm, and gazing warmly at her caregiver. She started the day with a string wrapped tightly around her arm. But when she approached the caregiver, she let him unravel it and let it fall to the floor. The third day was a marked improvement over the previous two. She readily entered the room and threw her string in the trash can. She participated for long periods of time and began to express her own warmth and affection more deeply, consistently, and naturally. Her caregiver was also warmer, more valuing, and more authentic. The transformation of each was intertwined with the other. Maxine showed no forms of self-injury, aggression, or withdrawal. On the contrary, she sought out engagement with him, began doing more and more on her own and in a more complex fashion, and actively sought the caregiver's affection.

What do Maxine and her caregiver teach us? Like many individuals, Maxine presented multiple challenges. The caregiver had to quickly learn how to designify the paranoid verbalizations, the string wrapped tightly around her arm, the attempts at biting herself and aggression toward himself, her fear of touch, her unwillingness to participate, and her running away. Much of the process of taking these old meanings away rested in his ability to give new meanings to being with him. He expressed strong feelings that she was safe with him by approaching her soothingly, by reaching toward her in a nonthreatening manner, and making sure that his words and touch were for valuing. At first, she approached him and rapidly spouted out, "She's coming! She's coming! The police woman is after me. I didn't do anything, but she's going to get me." A common caregiver response would be to explain that there is no police woman, asking her to realize this, and trying to enable the expression of a logical and reasoned thought process. However, a person in an incoherent and driven mood responds very poorly to reasoning since their thoughts are by nature disorganized. In order to make the police woman "disappear," the caregiver had to pay it no heed and yet assure her that she was safe. This cognitive-emotional resignification process involves a turning of thoughts and feelings to the here-and-now, the strong expression of the goodness of his presence, the ongoing elicitation of valuing from her, and deflecting the fixation as much as possible.

We need to be willing to deal with the constellation of challenges that the person presents by centering ourselves on a new relationship. The first several hours or weeks can be most difficult and our endurance is important. The process is wrought with a multiplicity of decisions: how we present ourselves, what we say, how we enable engagement, and which techniques to use. We have to be ready to respond to each of these and base our interactions on increased valuing and decreased domination.

Daniel

Daniel was a 50-year-old man with a diagnosis of mild retardation. He was unable to hear or verbally communicate, but could communicate with caregivers skilled in signing. He had a history of actively withdrawing from almost all interactions and preferred to be alone. He was noted for his rigidity, especially obvious in an unwillingness to deviate from his routines, which included a ritual of drinking coffee after any act of "compliance," followed by chewing tobacco. If he did not receive these "rein-forcers," he would rush toward his caregivers and demand them by flailing his arms and making loud sounds. At these times, he would also bang his wrists against his chest and head. When not satisfied, he would also use strong physical force to attain his desired end.

His emotional appearance was markedly sad. He had a flat affect, seldom smiled, and rarely reached out toward others in a warm way. His caregivers described him as high-strung, tactilely defensive, rebellious toward strangers, and easily upset. As a defense mechanism, he had learned to run away from them when-ever he was told to do something. To deal with this, they had habituated him to a "behavioral contract" that involved receiving coffee and tobacco for compliance with their demands. He would not deviate from this rigidly fixed routine without acts of aggres-sion or running away. Although this behavioral truce achieved some control, it left him as a solitary person with no friendships and coffee and tobacco as the center of his emotional life. He was provided with a daily contract that indicated his schedule. He received tobacco and coffee for acts of obedience, and these were withheld for any deviations. For aggression, he was placed in a time-out room "until calm" and also failed to receive his con-tingent rewards for that hour. He was physically restrained for more severe aggression. When he destroyed any property, he would have to repeatedly clean up the mess that he had made. He would generally follow his mandated contract, but still acted out if he "felt stress." More significantly, his caregivers reported that, although these strategies had an immediate impact in terms of generating obedience, his relationship with them was deteriorat-ing and he was becoming a more distancing person.

When a caregiver resolved to enter a mutual change process with Daniel, the initial hours necessitated the mobilization of a number of strategies capable of enabling participation since he was fearful, distancing, and disengaging. Plus, he was now accustomed to contingent reward. Any physical proximity on the caregiver's part brought movement away. If asked to do something, he would either do it obligatorily or run away. He expected his coffee and tobacco for any deed done. His caregiver decided to make it a non-issue by "legalizing" it, but also continuing to bring about participation. The running away was partially resolved by greeting him kindly prior to his entrance, having his work area well-prepared, and being flexible if he refused to participate immediately. Since Daniel could not hear and was also tactilely defensive, value-giving had to be expressed warmly through gestures. Despite his hearing problem and fear of being touched, he also was expected to learn to accept physical valuing in the form of handshakes. At first, the caregiver just touched his hand. The first such contacts were presented quickly and with as little imposition as possible. As the hours unfolded, he began to willingly accept this and then initiate it in the form of smiles, gazing, and handshakes. On several occasions, he swung his arms at the caregiver and then ran to another area when he no longer wanted to participate. However, his aggression appeared to be more out of fear than anger, so his caregiver concentrated on signalling safety and security rather than any force. As he participated more, his caregiver began to notice less fear and rebellion. After a week, he no longer ran from the caregiver. He was willing to spend lengthy periods of time working with the caregiver and sharing handshakes, pats on the back, and other forms of valuing. His behavioral contract for compliance had lost its meaning and was replaced by his new relationship with a particular caregiver.

What do Daniel and his caregiver teach us? A mechanistic approach toward behavioral change might bring about a behavioral stalemate, but we need to ask whether a sterile emotional world is worth this. A critical question in the life of someone who is disconnected from feelings of mutuality is, "What sentiments are conveyed through the scheduled delivery of material rewards?" Daniel and his caregiver had to pass through a process of establishing feelings of safety, security, engagement, and valuing. These had to become more powerful than the materialistic attraction of coffee and tobacco. Their "leglization" helped remove them as a battle ground and enabled a focus on building a relationship. However, many find it intolerable to "give in" to something that should be "earned." We need to model this alternative approach and help other caregivers question their purpose.

Daniel's major barriers to change involved his difficulty in communicating, his fear of his caregivers, and his life based on contingent reward. His emotional well-being had been worsened by his inability to reach out and the reluctance of those around him to bring him into their world. We need to understand that when a person is disconnected from these feelings of union, words alone cannot make up for this emptiness. The person has to feel our total authenticity. As Daniel started to sense this, he began to come closer. Initially, fear was a central aspect of life. The caregiver's touch and gestures had to communicate safety and human valuing and transform the fear into a desire to be with the caregiver. At first, this made no sense. However, the more the caregiver expressed this, the less fearful and more comfortable Daniel became. Finally, the caregiver had to counteract Daniel's long history of a life based on a behavioral contract. He expected contingent reward, this had been hammered into him. The caregiver had to be tolerant enough to designify this part of his life by making the coffee and tobacco available to him at any time, whether earned or not. However, the key was to simultaneously bring about engagement and gradually replace the drive for material reward with unconditional valuing and human engagement.

BEYOND OURSELVES

Some might think, "This is fine. You have changed your relationship. What about everyone else?" These feelings do not transfer from one person to another. We have a responsibility to spread them outward. It is always better to start with two or three others. But, if this is impossible, we can at least begin on our own. The individual teacher, although working with handicapped children far removed from the mainstream, can begin with one child, then her assistant, and then other children. She can invite a teacher-friend to talk about changing their grassroots reality. Over

---

Going Beyond Individual Change

- Define a clear picture of reality: our values and actions, the world in which we work or live, the person's world, the values and practices of other caregivers.
- Bring as many others into the process as possible: model your interactions, share your values, help others form feelings of companionship.
- Create cultural circles among these small groups: meet frequently, examine relationships, define purposes, identify oppressive policies and practices, make personal and group commitments.
- Expand the number of individuals interested in a mutual change process.

---

time, their small group can transform one classroom, then two. The single parent can begin helping his child. There might not seem to be enough time, yet this parent can initiate the process through new interactions and structuring time so that a new pattern begins to take hold. This parent can then invite other parents and teachers into the change process. Regardless of our reality, we need to begin with ourselves and then create small groups of like-minded others. It might not seem like much, but these circles of others can start to change reality. They are like yeast in dough: a small amount of change can gradually transform the mass.

CONCLUSION

"What you can try if . . ." can be posed in thousands of ways with thousands of responses. We have only examined a few. What we need to remember is that our values are the key in any of these challenging situations. In the first dimension, establishing a spirit of companionship depends on subtle aspects of our interactions. It is important to feel confident that there is an evolving solidarity in spite of highly disruptive interactions. None of the questions has a simple answer. Each one involves a dynamic process between the caregiver and the person that is ever-changing. How we might respond to any given situation is highly personal and fluid. These suggestions and examples are only intended to give some insight as to how our posture toward the person leads us to become teachers of valuing and engagement. The driving force in our decisions has to be centered in our option for a culture of life, questioning reality, and moving toward companionship. When in doubt, we should opt for valuing and dialogue. Whether in the "What if . . .?" questions or the specific examples, our central role is unconditional valuing. We cannot deviate from this if we want to establish companionship. The process asks much of us. The initial focus is on us, not on changing the other person. However, as we begin to change and draw more closely to marginalized people, our task is to bring others along to form circle of friends and change reality.

Chapter 10
COMING HOME

We have tried to describe the inner feelings of those who cannot speak for themselves: those silenced by domination, slowed by mental handicap, disturbed by mental illness, and bowed by the ravages of poverty and the lack of opportunity to feel one with others. Yet hope and resilience abide as they withstand isolation, seclusion, chemicals, restraint, and punishment. Few of us could resist so many years of oppression and human denial. Few could tolerate programs and services endowed with a pathology of compliance and a fetish for "appropriate" behaviors. To be marginalized is more than a clinical status; it is a social condition in which people are pushed and pulled to the outer edges of community, to a point so distant that it is no longer community. Prejudice, categorizations, and technology are the instruments that force people to this extremity of the human condition. They are pushed with cattle prods or pulled with restraint devices. Or, more commonly, their hope is taken away by someone's distancing words, cold touch, and empty gaze. We then wonder why their aggression is so severe, their self-injury so violent, or their withdrawal so deep.

THE MARGINALIZED

It is a pity that Magdalene, a young woman in a masked helmet in the South, cannot speak. She would look at us with a despairing gaze; her eyes would scan the surrounding movements through her black-wire-mesh world like a prisoner within her own entombing cell. If we were to look through the wire mask, we would see scars and sorrow marking her retreat from others into a domain of solitude where her only joy arises from self-mutilation. But hope always lives, even though it is sometimes buried deeply. It is a pity that she cannot speak when she is unmasked, the doorway of her loneliness swinging open, the helmet falling to the terrazzo floor, and her eyes looking upward for one brief moment in silent thanksgiving—a life of tears and abandonment about to be transformed into a life of meaning and union. This is the hope of interdependence.

It is a shame that the Pig-Boy, a child of the Americas, cannot speak—a child found among the pigs in a city dump, eating the town's garbage, protected by the swine and other abandoned children. He would tell us so much about the world in which our excess is tossed in the city's dump—about the food, the bottles, the bags, and the children. This child, if only he could speak, would relate how a 3-year-old survives, along with other defenseless ones, with the comradeship of pigs. He would also tell us how one day he was found and placed in the city's asylum. He would recall how he sat with his head cast downward, with his little hands tied to the sides of a wooden chair. The Pig-Boy would share his dreams about the leftover life of those who are abandoned, the nights accompanied by the warm bodies of the pigs, the meaning of life heard in their grunts and snorts and felt in the putrid stench of fetid food. If we were to look at him, he would teach us much: tolerance of the defenseless, empathy for those who are voiceless, and authenticity toward those who seem to have nothing to give. It is a pity that he cannot now speak when his hands are finally freed, his body cared for, and his heart warmed. He would surely tell us long stories with the touch of his arms around our waiting hearts. With a smile, he would lift up his child-body and would seek out the one who freed him and who now gives warmth instead of coldness. How powerful is the hunger for union in the face of abandonment!

It is a pity that Nora cannot rise up. She speaks, but nobody listens. Her shattered hallucinatory words are beyond the grasp of those who cannot feel. She finds solace only in tearing her skin from her delicate face now pocked with the years of self-mutilation brought about by meaninglessness, aloneness, and choicelessness. Some say she is insane and that the condition of schizophrenia drives her to harm herself. Yet, when approached, she smiles and teases. She only becomes angry when she is left alone in the dark corner of the asylum's seclusion room. Perhaps it is the nature of her insanity to dig her fingernails into her face, yet one wonders why she is so affectionate when others give her warm love. It is a pity that she cannot just leave through the locked doors and barred windows since she would surely find someone to be at home with. So often, we are the bars, the chicken-wire windows, and the locked doors. It is our hearts that need to be unlocked and opened so that mutual freedom might be possible.

These are the people who are incarcerated, abandoned, and subjugated, or they are the ones who become their caregivers' companions. Each is marginalized. Many are born vulnerable to social isolation due to mental retardation, mental illness, or other disabilities. Yet people stand with their arms folded and shove the marginalized further away instead of drawing themselves toward them. To be marginalized is to be alone in the midst of others. It is to be fearful in the presence of others. It is to rebel at cold demands and seek attention through self-harm. It is to attack in the face of domination or to give up in the shadow of despair. It is a life based on the expectation of compliance and one devoid of warmth. It is a life based on reward and punishment and one ripped from any feelings of companionship and interdependence.

The Marginalizers

And what about us? We take no joy in this dispirited human condition. We know that each marginalized person is a mirror image of ourselves and that, when we look closely, their anguish is ours and their hope is ours. Most of us have had at least momentary feelings of apartness, even if not of being marginalized and infringed upon as much as those whom we serve. Yet some of us still carry out jail-like plans: the locking of doors, the distribution of drugs, the shocking with cattle prods, the escorting to this room or that room. Or, while some do these deeds, others sit in their coffee-stained offices devising new plans with better contingencies for the robopaths under their charge. A glance at programs and services can open our eyes. Walk into a school and witness a teacher staring disinterestedly at the children. Open a front door and watch a parent spank a child. Listen to the group home caregiver make fun of the almost helpless person. Walk by a nurse in a hospital and listen to the mockery, "We ought to put her in the lock-up ward!" Walk through the slums and city streets, go into a shelter, and sit next to the homeless men and women as they hold the tattered photographs of love long lost.

To marginalize is to participate in acts of social injustice. It is often the moment-to-moment deeds done without any consideration of the wholeness of the other: It is our drive to achieve obedience in a world devoid of friendship; it is our boredom with the person and our fascination with their behaviors; it is not only our fixation on efficient programs, planing, and data, but also our blindness to the person's feelings and their human condition; it is our self-degradation. If we cannot see the full humanity of the other person, we cannot see it in ourselves.

Fortunately, even in the midst of oppression, men and women of values emerge—rejecting a culture of death and seeking out ways to give life and hope—some quietly, some loudly, some behind closed doors, some publicly. Each of us is challenged to assume a posture of solidarity, to break away from acts of marginalization, and to rupture the culture of death. Caregiving is an act of social justice, the instillation of hope, and entering a journey toward home. It is the teacher who befriends the slow or recalcitrant child. It is the tired parent who stays awake in the night and gives affection to the crying child. It is the group home caregiver who welcomes the stranger and makes friendship. It is the nurse who stays with the frightened patient. It is the advocate who sits and shares a meal with the homeless person.

Alison looks at Magdalene enshrouded in her helmet—hardly able to see her face, let alone her forlorn eyes. But Alison looks, stays, and takes her hand. Her serenity in the face of daily struggle is only overshadowed by the affection that she holds for Magdalene as she touches her hand. Alison removes the helmet and cares for the child as if she were her own. Without a doubt, it is difficult since there is so much to do and so little time. Nevertheless, she knows that each moment of giving has precious meaning. Eyes open. Faces soften. Hands reach out.

Maria looks warmly at the Pig-Boy, now christened Panchito. She is working in the asylum for the abandoned and has watched him being tied to a chair since his arrival in the psychiatric hospital, his frail arms restrained with pink ribbons to prevent him from slamming his head onto the floor. One day, she resolves to treat him with the love and tenderness of a mother. She dares to untie him, hold him, and play with him. Her words initially seem to make no sense and her grasp seems to bring fear. Day after day, she reaches out toward him, and then one day he suddenly lifts up his head, touches her face, and embraces her. Love reciprocates love.

And likewise, Gaston begins to listen to Nora's expressions. He hears her words of despair. Moving carefully, he approaches her. She screams and tries to hit and gouge her face. He places his hands to protect her scarred face. She scratches him, but she also looks at him. He tries to teach her not to fear him, not to sense domination and mandates, but the giving of affection and value. The days wear on. Gaston begins to feel more at ease as she becomes less intense in her rejection, even sometimes smiling and beckoning him to her. Both seem to know that they have entered into a process of mutual change.

We can refuse to marginalize. We can elect to become companions. The establishment of justice knows no limits if dialogue is at the center.

Our challenge is to reflect on and practice a psychology of human interdependence wherein feelings of safety and security replace those of fear and loathing; the feeling of being with the other replaces the absurdity of isolation and withdrawal; and the expression of unconditional valuing overcomes the driven desires for compliance, obedience, and control.

> Brian reaches out to Mary, his adopted child, only to receive deep scratches in return. He does not coil in fear or retribution. He stays by her side. He soothes rather than yells; he values rather than castigates. At first, she runs, screams, and flails her arms. But Brian approaches and reaches out. The child's fingernails gouge deeply into his outstretched arms. She stops and looks as if asking herself whether he will retaliate or endure. For a split second, she pauses and almost smiles. Brian stays with her. He knows his commitment is to give value to her and someday she will give it back. And that day comes with amazing haste, for Mary's heart, like everyone's, longs for feelings of being at home.

A STRUGGLE WITHIN AND WITHOUT

Interdependence is a psychology of life in which we recognize that we all long for union and a feeling of being at home in spite of the crusted layers of ice that sometimes cover our hearts. The warmth that thaws this ice is what we can bring to the emergent relationship with the marginalized person. Just as those whom we serve, we have an inner hope to be one with others, but at the same time harbor a fear of self-surrender. Likewise, we struggle with those around us in a battle between domination and union. It is a difficult life-project that requires mutual change since it is not only the other person who is emotionally frozen. This can befall all who walk the face of the earth. As caregivers, we have a special responsibility to recognize the meaning of the human condition and procure ways to reveal and express the feeling of being at home while bring the warmth of companionship to those who await it. No change in the other will transpire until it occurs in us. We are the ones who need the commitment to reach out. But this extension of self cannot occur until we begin to question our values and put them into practice. Our inner struggle between the fear of giving and the hope of companionship is where we need to start. It is felt with uneasiness. It is a process in which we need to constantly engage ourselves with marginalized people, persevere in the difficult moments of rejection, and know that mutual change will come. Ongoing battles between the urge for compliance and the pursuit of companionship symbolize this inner struggle. We are confronted with institutionalized violence, whose cold blood circulates through service programs. We have to ask ourselves which is our role: to dominate or to value? If we opt for the latter, we then choose to enter into a process of human interdependence.

This struggle is within us all, such as in the case of Lisa and her mother. Frustrated by the nonresponsiveness of her daughter, the mother begins to feel that perhaps punishment will modify her child's behavior in a "spare-the-rod, spoil-the-child" spirit. She proceeds to enter into a domineering relationship. The stubborn child throws her meal on the floor or has a temper tantrum, and the mother follows her new plan, mustering up the energy to yell, "No!" If the tossing or crying continues, she repeats the ultimatum. If it does not work, she then holds her child's hands down for ten seconds. What had been instruments of love now become tools of oppression.

Yet, the mother begins to feel troubled and struggles with her new role of domination. Lisa fights with her and often resists the reprimands. What the mother sees as firmness, the child perceives as mean-spirited. She sometimes obeys, but obedience is unlike love since it arises out of a spirit of control. Lisa's heart is becoming fearful and the mother feels that frigidity is replacing warmth. Both are becoming less.

One day the mother has had enough. She begins to reflect on her love for her daughter. She looks at their crumbling relationship and chooses to return to nurturing. She asks herself, "Why not teach Lisa to share and to come to me because I love her? To feel that love is mutual? To accept my warmth and learn to give it back?" She sits with her child and starts to teach her to share. She dialogues with her, "You give Mommy your doll, and I will give it

right back. Lisa, it is good to be with me. I want to be with you!"
At first, the child is perplexed. The dialogue does not immediately
translate into feelings of warmth and affection. She sometimes
smiles, then rebels, and smiles once more. Love and respect start
to take hold. The mother continues to nurture Lisa even when she
refuses to share and throws the doll on the floor: "Mommy will
help you more. Just for a second. Now here it is!" The journey
back home is hard, but the mother perseveres. She hands her the
doll and asks for it in return. All the while, she talks with the child
about feelings of friendship, love, and sharing. When the child
becomes momentarily recalcitrant, she does not grimace, yell, or
use force; rather, she continues the giving and receiving process
interwoven with warm words. As time passes, Lisa and her mother
begin to sense a deepening union. Smiles emerge and words become warmer. Mother and child have started to return to a culture
of life.

The outer struggle is most often found in our urge to express
our fears through controlling others and the mobilization of a tool
box filled with a variety of institutionalized, culturally acceptable
practices. Lisa's mother felt lost and fearful. She had given up the
hopefulness of her nurturing and had fallen into the ritual of
compliance. The trappings of control are wrought with tempting
facades. Data is easily produced to validate violence's power. Prescribed plans embellish the process. Special buildings are erected
to perform the more esoteric rites. Yet, as with Lisa's mother, the
question gnaws away: "What am I doing to my child?" And, more
frequently than not, hope overcomes fear and nonviolence is
stronger than force.

Last Words

Each of us is on a journey. Some move along the road with
more ease and comfort. Like all journeys, there are detours and
barriers. Some become lost; others are not certain of where they
are going. All of us need direction and help, some more than

others. This life project requires purposefulness defined and questioned, and it calls for endurance and patience. It is always wiser to move in the company of others, for during the dark nights of the spirit, it is safer and more secure to be with those whom we love than to be alone. Nobody wants to be pushed or dragged down this road. Nobody chooses to wander aimlessly. But everyone can become lost whether it be Lisa's momentary parallel life with her mother, Magdalene's masked existence, the Pig-Boy's abandonment, Nora's retreat into unreality, or Mary's violence. Coming together makes the road less dangerous, less lonely, and less detoured. It is what can guide us home.

The feeling of being at home is much more than the arrival at a destination; it is the journey itself. It is the companionship of others and their support throughout life. It is warmth on the cold days of the spirit and hands united during stormy moments. It is laughter and tears. It is an ongoing and expanding coming together. It is not merely the strong helping the weak, nor the fast accompanying the slow. It has nothing to do with charity; it has to do with the struggle for union through justice. Coming home is the process of the human condition. It is not a point at which we ever arrive; rather, it is the horizon toward which we move and on the way gather others. And this gathering helps the dawn move closer.

The purpose of caregiving is a life-long project that leads Alison to accompany Magdalene in the difficult task of protecting her while also bringing about a new spirit wherein the slamming of the head in anguish is replaced by the smile of human warmth. It leads Maria to loosen and eventually untie the pink ribbons from Panchito's arms and teach him and herself to give. It leads Nora's caregiver to replace hallucinations with dialogue. It leads Brian to tolerate Mary's lashing out while at the same time transforming hits and scratches into reaching out. It leads Lisa's mother to see Lisa in need of learning to both receive and to give.

To give care is to instill hope, to question and change reality, and to form a life of companionship. Throughout the world, children and adults by the hundreds of thousands live apart. Some have been abandoned out of hopelessness. Others live in hunger imposed by unjust social and economic structures. Others are scooped up and placed in multi-million dollar warehouses. Others are segregated like lepers. And some are lost at home. Yet, as caregivers, we are asked to enter these worlds and generate feelings of friendship and justice with one, then two, and then untold numbers of those who are marginalized.

Panchito lived in a world caved in by the weight of personal, political, and economic abandonment. Yet, one caregiver, Maria, was able to begin to bring him and others hope. She knew, like we do, that she had to enter a life-long project with him and eventually find ways to help other nameless children. Like Maria, our challenge is to enter the darkened world of the abandoned, the forgotten, and the segregated. Maria's struggle is perhaps more difficult than many caregivers', but we can begin to accompany her and Panchito with those whom we serve. Her reality was one of near hopelessness yet she instilled hope. It was one of abandonment, yet she brought companionship. Let us end this book feeling what Maria and Panchito felt.

> Christ, atop the highest hill,
> Looks upon the city,
> Arms of stone opened
> Toward the housed and the fed,
> Eyes fixed firmly
> On the land of the living.
>
> The sun shines on His face,
> Casting a cascading shadow
> Behind and down the darkened hillside,
> Impacting on white tombstones,
> Each rising from the ground
> Like rectangular scars.
>
> At the bottom,
> On the opposite side of the Street of Tears,
> On the darkened plain,
> The earth has opened up,

Pushing out a tomb for the abandoned,
For twenty-seven children
Frozen between life and death,
Chilled by the lengthening shadow,
Forgotten by the fattened city dwellers
On the other side of the hill.

Child Salvador,
Body black,
Arms outstretched,
Approached,
Sucking a red plastic cord,
His lips never having touched
A mother's breast.

Juan Luis,
Pale face,
Eyes moving from side to side
Like rounded ice,
Stands alone,
Frozen in time,
An infant child
Imagining what he has never seen.

Claudia
Sits on a wooden stool,
Lips moving,
Whispering, crying,
"Come, come, come!"
Words not answered.

And Panchito,
Head cast downward,
Rocks himself,
His blinded eyes fixed
On his tiny strapped arms
Listening to an unsung song.

And twenty-three others
Are twisted images of these four.

Though named,
They are nameless.
Though gowned,
They are naked.
Though living,
They are dead.
Until someone is touched
By the twenty-seven.

Maria, warm-hearted,
In the midst of coldness,
Reaches down,
Unties Panchito,
And lifts him up,
The beginning of the instillation
Of hope.

Each of us is called on to walk into these worlds. Some glisten with ceramic tiles. Some reek with odors. We do not want to live in a culture of death, but one of life. Like Maria, we can reach into these tombs of nothingness, refuse to opt for the darkness of the night, and help create human interdependence. And one day our Panchito will look warmly at us, reach his hands out, and embrace us.

SUGGESTED READINGS

Biklen, D. P. (1983). *Community organizing: Theory and practice.* Englewood Cliffs, NJ: Prentice-Hall.

Bowlby, J. (1969). *Attachment and love.* London: Hogarth.

Buber, M. (1965). *Between man and man.* New York: Macmillan.

Buber, M. (1970). *I and thou.* New York: Charles Scribner.

Campbell, P. (1987). *Use of aversive procedures with persons who are disabled: An historical review and critical analysis.* Seattle, WA: The Association for Persons with Severe Handicaps.

Carr, E. G., & Durand, V. M. (1986). The social-communicative basis of severe behavior problems in children. In S. Reiss & R. Bootuzi (Eds.), *Theoretical issues in behavior therapy.* New York: Academic Press.

Carr, E. G., & McDowell, J. J. (1980). Social control of self-injurious behavior of organic etiology. *Behavior Therapy, 11,* 402–409.

Carr, E. G., Newsom, C. D., & Binkoff, J. A. (1976). Stimulus control of self-destructive behavior in a psychotic child. *Journal of Abnormal Child Psychology, 4,* 139–153.

Donnellan, A. M., Mirenda, P. L., Mesaros, R. A., & Fassbender, L. L. (1984). Analyzing the communicative functions of aberrant behavior. *Journal of the Association for Persons with Severe Handicaps, 9*(3), 201–212.

Durand, V. M., & Carr, E. G. (1987). Social influences on "self-stimulatory" behavior: Analysis and treatment application. *Journal of Behavior Analysis, 20*(2), 119–132.

Eisler, R. (1987). *The chalice and the blade: Our history, our future.* New York: Harper & Row.

Favell, J. E., Azrin, N. H., Baumeister, A. A., Carr, E. G., Dorsey, M. F., Lovass, O. I., Rincover, A., Risley, T. R., Romanczy, K. R. G., Russo, D. C., Schroeder, S. R., & Solnick, J. V. (1982). The treatment of self-injurious behavior. *Behavior Therapy, 13,* 529–554.

Fehrenbach, P. A., & Thelen, M. H. (1982). Behavioral approaches to the treatment of aggressive disorders. *Behavior Modification, 6*(4), 465–497.

Foucault, M. (1979). *Discipline and punish: The birth of the prison.* New York: Vintage Books.

Foucault, M. (1987). *Mental illness and psychology.* Berkley, CA: University of California Press.

Freire, P. (1970). *The pedagogy of the oppressed.* New York: Continuum.

Freire, P. (1973). *Education for critical consciousness.* New York: Continuum.

Fromm, E. (1973). *The anatomy of human destructiveness.* New York: Holt, Rinehart and Winston.

Gorman-Smith, D., & Matson, J. L. (1985). A review of treatment research for self-injurious and stereotyped responding. *Journal of Mental Deficiency Research, 29,* 295–308.

Johnson, W. L., & Baumeister, A. A. (1978). Self-injurious behavior: A review and analysis of methodological details of published studies. *Behavior Modification, 2,* 465–487.

Jordan, J., Singh, N. N., & Repp, A. (1989). An evaluation of gentle teaching and visual screening in the reduction of stereotypy. *Journal of Applied Behavior Analysis, 22*(1), 9–22.

LaGrow, S. J., & Repp, A. D. (1984). Stereotypic responding: A review of intervention research. *American Journal of Mental Deficiency, 88,* 595–609.

Laing, R. D. (1969). *Self and others.* New York: Pantheon Books.

Laing, R. D. (1969). *The divided self: An existential study in sanity and madness,* New York: Penguin Books.

Lavigna, G. W., & Donnellan, A. M. (1986). *Alternatives to punishment: Solving behavior problems with non-aversive strategies.* New York: Irvington.

Lovass, O. I., Newsom, C., & Hickman, C. (1987). Self-stimulatory behavior and perceptual reinforcement. *Journal of Applied Behavior Analysis, 20,* 45–68.

Lovett, H. (1985). *Cognitive counseling and persons with special needs: Adapting behavioral approaches to the social context.* New York: Praeger.

McGee, J. (1989). *Being with others: Toward a psychology of human interdependence.* Omaha, NE: Creighton University.

McGee, J. J., & Menolascino, F. J. (1990). Depression in persons with mental retardation: Toward an existential perspective. In A. Dosen

& F. J. Menolascino (Eds.), *Depression in mentally retarded children and adults* (95–112), Amsterdam: PAOS–Leiden.

McGee, J. J., & Menolascino, F. J. (in press). The impact of gentle teaching on a child with life threatening self-injurious behavior. In W. Stainback (Ed.), *Controversial perspectives*. New York: Allyn & Bacon.

McGee, J., Menolascino, F. J., Hobbs, D. C., & Menousek, P. E. (1987). *Gentle teaching: A non-aversive approach to helping persons with mental retardation*. New York: Human Sciences Press.

McGee, J. J. (1990). Gentle teaching: The basic tenet. *Nursing Times, 86,* (2), 68–72.

Menolascino, F. J., & McGee, J. J. (1983). Persons with severe mental retardation and behavioral challenges: From disconnectedness to human engagement. *Journal of Psychiatric Treatment and Evaluation, 5,* 187–193.

Meyer, L. H., & Evans, I. M. (1989). *Non-aversive intervention for behavior problems: A Manual for home and community*. Baltimore: Paul H. Brookes.

Montagu, A., & Matson, F. (1983). *The dehumanization of man*. New York: McGraw-Hill.

Mudford, O. C. (1985). Treatment selection in behavior reduction: Gentle teaching vs. the least intrusive treatment model. *Australia and New Zealand Journal of Developmental Disabilties, 10,* 265–270.

O'Donnell, J. M. (1985). *The origins of behaviorism: American psychology, 1870–1920*. New York: New York University Press.

Rincover, A. (1986). Behavioral research in self-injury and self-stimulation. *Psychiatric Clinics of North America, 9*(4), 755–765.

Rincover, A., & Devany, J. (1982). The application of sensory extinction procedures to self-injury. *Analysis and Intervention in Developmental Disabilities, 3,* 67–81.

Rioux, M. H. (1988). *The language of pain: Perspectives on behavior management*. Toronto: The G. Allan Roeher Institute.

Schor, I., & Freire, P. (1987). *A pedagogy for liberation: Dialogues on transforming education*. South Hadley, MA: Bergin and Garvey Publishers.

Sroufe, L. A., & Waters, E. (1977). *The ontogenesis of smiling and laughter: A perspective on the organization of development in infancy. Psychological Review, 83* (3), 173–189.

Teodoro, G., & Barrera, S. J. (1989). An experimental analysis of gentle teaching: *Clinical Bulletin of the Developmental Disabilities Program of the University of Western Ontario, 1,* 3.

Unger, R. M. (1984). *Passion: An essay on personality.* New York: The Free Press.
Yalom, I. D. (1980). *Existential psychotherapy.* New York: Basic Books.
Watzlawick, P., Beavin, J., & Jackson, D. (1967). *The pragmatics of human communication.* New York: W. W. Norton.

INDEX

227

Printed in the United States
50898LVS00001B/136